GW01459118

A guide to
Phototherapy Practice
Theory and Underpinning Science

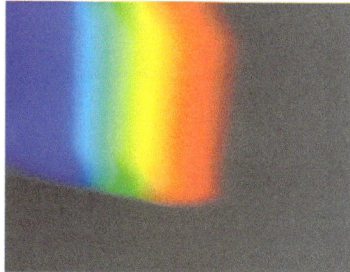

A guide to
Phototherapy Practice

Theory and Underpinning Science

Dr David C Somerville PhD CSci FRSA

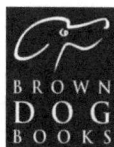

BROWN
DOG
BOOKS

Copyright © David Somerville 2017

The right of David Somerville to be identified as the author of this work has been asserted in accordance with the Copyright, Designs & Patents Act 1988.

All rights reserved. No part of this book may be reproduced, stored in a retrieval system, or transmitted in any form or by any means, electronic, electrostatic, magnetic tape, mechanical, photocopying, recording or otherwise, without the written permission of the copyright holder.

Published under licence by Brown Dog Books and
The Self-Publishing Partnership, 7 Green Park Station, Bath BA1 1JB

www.selfpublishingpartnership.co.uk

ISBN printed book 978-1-78545-211-6
e-book 978-1-78545-212-3

Cover design by Kevin Rylands
Internal design by Andrew Easton

Printed and bound by CPI Group (UK) Ltd, Croydon CR0 4YY

Dedicated to my wife Marjorie for her understanding, patience and assistance in writing this book.

Thanks go to Professor Mark Lythgoe, University College London, for papers provided and permission for the use of an illustration taken from his research into photo-acoustics.

Also, thanks go to veterinary physiotherapists Anne Upson, Tomos Garbett-Davies and Emma Sellars for their case history reports and photos.

Foreword

This is the second book in a series looking at specific electrotherapies by the same author. The first one was titled: 'A Guide to Pulsed Magnetic Therapy and Underpinning Science'. These books arise out of requests from students, practitioners and owners of various electrotherapy units and applicators. The two most commonly requested are phototherapy and pulsed magnetic therapy. The author has worked alongside therapists for over 20 years, has a doctorate in clinical orthopaedic research and was trained in electronics and avionics engineering in the Royal Air Force. He studied for an honours degree in physical sciences and education before embarking on his medical research studies. Post-doctoral studies included research into non-invasive therapies used to treat orthopaedic problems and soft tissue effects. In 1995, he was asked to give a lecture on pulsed magnetic therapy to a small group of therapists. Since then he has lectured around the world on the use of pulsed magnetism and phototherapy to both human and animal physiotherapists and helped set up courses in veterinary physiotherapy as well as being a founder member of the Institute of Registered Veterinary and Animal Physiotherapists (IRVAP).

This book follows a logical sequence and develops the science and theory behind light production and its biological effects. It also includes some interesting and possibly original theories. The science is logically developed and uses analogies from the author's background in electronics and avionics to deliver an all-round grounding in the subject.

Notes

Contents

Introduction 12

1. Safety Considerations 15

2. Phototherapy Application and Dosage 21

3. The Science Underpinning Light Production 37

4. Photons; The Enigmatic Entity 47

5. LASERs (it's all done by mirrors!) 55

6. Absorption Characteristics into Tissue 66

7. The Basics of Cellular Biology 80

8. A Resonance Theory of Cellular Interactions 86

9. The Research 96

10. Case Histories 108

11. Summary and Conclusions 117

Bibliography and References 121

List of illustrations

Figure	Content
1.	Blocking colours ring
2.	Spectral radiance output of the sun
3.	Treatment points along a sutured wound
4.	Applicator Treatment around an open wound
5.	Typical illustration of a carbon atom
6.	Oxygen molecule
7.	Carbon dioxide molecule
8.	Sub level references orbitals
9.	Visible part of the electromagnetic spectrum
10.	Simplified view of electron stimulation and energy release
11.	A theory of photon emission process
12.	Electron stimulation between energy levels
13.	Ruby laser
14.	P-N Junction LASER diode
15.	Fabry-Perot resonant cavity
16.	Photons as waves 'in step'
17.	Light emitting diode (SLD) used in therapy
18.	A Steradian (radius squared)
19.	Light emitting diode symbol and circuitry
20.	Cluster of SLDs additive effect
21.	Energy attenuation in tissue (Baxter)
22.	Example of horizontal and vertical polarity in radio transmissions
23.	Comparison of laser and LED scatter patterns

24.   Beam comparisons using a less turbid medium

25.   Section of cell membrane phospholipid bi-layer structure

26.   Typical animal prokaryotic cell

27.   Simplified diagram of a tuned transmitter and receiver

28.   Simplified optical cone cell

29.   Prokaryotic bacterial cellular structure

30.   Phototherapy reactions within a cell

31.   Photoacoustic image showing blood vessels in a human hand

32.   Thermal image of Ben

33.   Anal furunculosis before and after treatment

34.   Photographic progress of horse injury after a car accident

35.   Photographic sequence -equine leg wound

List of tables

36.   Energy transfer timings for a single emitter covering 1cm2 under ideal conditions

37.   Recommended treatments for a variety of injuries

38.   Functions of organelles within eukaryotic cells

39.   Comparative frequency sensitivities for the three types of cone cells

Note: *All drawings are copyright to the author but are free to use for non-commercial education purposes.*

Introduction

Light generating technology has developed significantly over the last few decades. Lasers and super bright emitters and their beneficial effects on tissue are becoming now a mainstream therapy for a variety of conditions. Phototherapy is one aspect of the science of light interactions with biological structures, and there are many papers and theories that can be found highlighting such interactions, but a limited number of books. This book is aimed at those who wish to incorporate phototherapy into mainly animal practice and is possibly less analytically scientific in its approach than any of the earlier works. For the therapist, a good working knowledge of basic physics and cellular biology would be useful to gain an insight into some of the concepts involved. It will explore what are, in the main, anecdotal reports of its efficacy and look at some case histories that have followed through treatments and the methods employed. It will also revisit some physics of light formation and suggest some new and possibly original theories of photon absorption into biological structures. The development of light sources other than true lasers has led to a more cost-effective approach to treatment with less issues over safety although minimum standards need to be observed. The main aim of this book is therefore to provide a good grounding in the subject of phototherapy, providing the foundations for those who wish to study the subject further from a deeper physics and biological point of view.

It should also be added that, as a medical research scientist teaching electrotherapies, mainly to veterinary and physiotherapy students and practitioners for over two decades, I have never been happy just to take at face value statements such as 'how a therapy works for this or that injury or condition'. These statements may well be correct, but in this book, I have gone further than most to try to disseminate how the interactions of photons with cellular molecular structures take place to cause beneficial or other effects for different conditions. I have theorised as to why certain organelles appear to be able to absorb photonic energy more efficiently than others. In all aspects, when teaching electrotherapies, I have felt that if the therapist is able to give a logical explanation of how and why a modality works, is applied and its beneficial biological interactions, this can only enhance their standing as a professional both in the eyes of veterinary surgeons and their more enquiring clients.

Phototherapy may come in many guises. Everything from simple bright lights to colour therapy could be claimed to be part of it. What this book intends to carry out is to discern what might be described as the 'scientific' aspects of it to general claims based on more doubtful evidence for its efficacy or certain ways of application. It will look at light as an essential part of our environment within the visible spectrum, not just for visual but for therapy aspects that may include both. To begin to understand light one must look at an energy form, or rather a method of transmitting and receiving such energy.

To many, the concept of visible light being in fact invisible may be difficult to comprehend. It is the effect of light on our receptors, especially within the eyes, that gives visibility to objects that have light reflected from them. The transmission of light must be invisible otherwise we would not be able to focus or discern physical objects because light energy would blank out everything. Light in its many forms has, therefore, to be viewed for what it is, a transfer of energy from a source to a receptor via both absorption and reflections of objects it encounters. The use of light in therapy is again making use of an energy transfer into tissue.

The laws of conservation of energy make a very simple but profound statement that 'energy cannot be created or destroyed, only changed'. Such changes are known as transduction, that is, energy may start from an initial but eternal source and carry on ad infinitum by changing to other forms. If we take the energy from the theory of the 'big bang' as being a starting block and a transformation of energy from whatever existed before it, then all energy around today owes its origins to this relative starting point, including light. It is important to understand how light energy originates from all sources and the factors causing its production. Understanding this is a basic requirement to be able to study how this energy form may be useful in therapy and to understand its transformation from light to other forms of energy within tissue. This includes further transformations into other frequencies of light.

The early chapters of this book will identify safety issues and address phototherapy as a treatment modality, including considerations and calculations for treatment dosage. The book then progresses to look at the basic science of light production, including some theories, and how light is absorbed and scattered in tissue. It will also discuss the different forms of phototherapy devices, how they are made and the range of light frequencies they produce. The later chapters of the book will look at biological effects related to light frequency. This includes some new theories and future developments for using light diagnostically. It will also include both established and ongoing research along with sample case studies, these being mainly centred on animal patients.

Chapter One

SAFETY CONSIDERATIONS

At this stage, safety considerations should be addressed for all methods of applying therapeutic energy transfers and the parameters for their safe use. These are hopefully covered in the manuals provided with them. This book is primarily dedicated to electrical powered equipment, mainly leaned towards veterinary use of phototherapy. When treating animals, the working environment may not be clinically perfect for treatments, especially where such treatments are carried out in the open and possibly damp environments. Treatments for human patients both in hospitals and clinics usually require that the equipment is cleared by a medical physics department before use. In many veterinary practices, PAT (portable appliance testing) is carried out on a regular basis by suitably qualified and registered service organisations. The following is a simple common-sense approach that, if followed, should keep the therapist, client owner and patient safe as well as ensure good maintenance of the equipment.

Application of all electrotherapies needs some degree of training and support. The term 'Electrotherapy' applies to '*any therapy that derives its functional application from an electrical source*'. Most of the operational dangers found in older equipment are related to their supply i.e. mains electrical supply and correspondingly high voltages within the equipment. Such dangers in modern equipment have been alleviated in that both the source of power to 'drive' the equipment is now increasingly a battery, driven at much lower voltages, also overall power consumption within equipment is now much reduced. However, whether high voltage or a battery supply, certain precautions are necessary and in general apply to all electrotherapies.

An electric current will always pass through the path of least resistance. This applies to both high and low voltage sources of such currents. Current is measured in amperes, usually contracted to 'amps'. The amount of current passing through any material is a function of the voltage level applied and the resistance encountered.

A simple expression of Ohm's law is that:

Current = Voltage / Resistance or I = V/R where I is in Amps, V is in Volts and R is in Ohms.

This simply means that if the resistance between two electric terminals is very low and the voltage fixed as with a battery, then the current that would flow between them is correspondingly very high. It follows, therefore, that very high voltages produce proportionately high currents under the same conditions. It is obvious that any electrical equipment is designed to operate within specific parameters. These are usually listed as temperature range, general environment and sometimes the length of time applied for treatment.

With therapists or veterinary surgeons working with their animal patients, the environment can be at the extremes at which their equipment can function. If the equipment is of the older type being powered by mains voltage supply, then extra precautions need to be observed. Stables can be damp or very wet in some cases and keeping the equipment dry is paramount. Cables need to be clear of any animals as hooves and their metal shoes which can easily cut through the cable, causing several potentially fatal situations. Live wires bared on a wet floor will effectively allow a current to pass through the liquid or over the damp surface to an earth. This current could also pass through the therapist, owner or the animal under treatment with dire consequences. Urine is highly conductive and equipment should be in places where contamination is totally avoided, away from the animal and any splashes from urination. Even in the drier environment of a clinic, mains cables should be well out of the reach of the patient, particularly if they are young and teething. Chewing on such cables could prove fatal if carrying mains supply.

Common sense is really the key to safe usage where mains voltages are concerned but the following should always be adhered to:

1. Never work completely alone, always be within sight or earshot of another person.

2. Carry out a risk assessment before commencing treatment.

3. If, despite all safety considerations an electrical accident occurs to either a human or animal present, always:

   a) If possible, switch off the supply. If not possible, try to disconnect the victim from the source of current by using a dry wooden broom handle or other plastic   dry implement.

   b) Never try to manually push the victim away from the electrical current source by hand.

4. When the situation is brought under control, always seek medical attention.

Where battery powered equipment is used these can still present problems in animal environments. Batteries are designed to deliver relatively high currents from low voltages. The energy in Watts is equal to the battery voltage x the current in Amps ($P = I \times V$). Damp contamination or accidental shorting of these batteries can cause an extremely high current to flow along any path of least resistance, causing heat and possible ignition or melting of the equipment with obvious consequences. All good equipment should be fuse protected. If, for example, damp conditions cause the fuse to blow, you should never be tempted to solve the problem with a short-term fix using silver paper or strands of wire. Seek professional assessment of the equipment and do not use until an all-clear has been given.

This book is specifically written for the subject of phototherapy. However, any equipment used either separately or at the same time needs the safety aspect to be considered. Good practice throughout will probably allow a long life for both the therapist, patient and equipment. Phototherapy comes with additional safety concerns regarding exposure not only to the eyes but over-exposure to tissue. Suitable glasses are recommended when using different frequencies. Red phototherapy can be effectively attenuated to visually safe levels with green glasses. Blue phototherapy needs yellow glasses. If infrared is used, then deep violet coloured type lenses would be needed, although very low powered devices may be screened by dark sunglasses.

High power infrared equipment being introduced comes with its own safety requirements regarding total screening of both the laser device and screening from the target area due to reflections. Whichever frequency or device power is used, care must also be taken in minimising reflections, especially when treating weeping wounds. With animals, owners need to be protected as well as the animal and therapist. A case was reported to me regarding visible red phototherapy where a well-known and experienced therapist decided to treat her own shoulder with a cluster device rated at a total overall output of 60milliWatts (60mW). Positioning it over the target area whilst sitting down, she fell asleep with the applicator still active. When she awoke she had a burn on the targeted area. It should be noted that the applicator delivered about 5mW per square centimetre for the exposure period but the affect accumulated to dangerous levels over the prolonged exposure.

Figure 1 below is used to illustrate a general principle that a filter that is pure green will only allow green wavelengths to pass through. A pure red wavelength would be completely absorbed by the filter. Caution should be taken both with infrared and ultra violet where they are to be applied. A deep violet screen in the form of glasses would reduce infrared-red. Higher frequencies in the ultraviolet wavebands may be screened by clear glass, not clear plastic. Safety glasses used in the most common colours are not necessarily pure green or yellow to allow a little observation of the treatment colour, but should be sufficient to filter down to safe observation levels. Extending this further into tissue, red pigmented tissue that appears red to the eye will accept and hence absorb all other colours and allow the red to pass through. Plants that rely on photosynthesis, if exposed to only green light, will have stunted growth and possibly die off. Green passes through or is reflected, all other colours are absorbed.

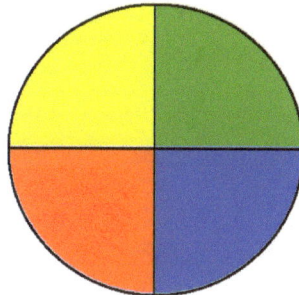

Figure 1. The basic blocking or 'anti colours' used in red and blue phototherapy shown diametrically opposite each other.

Equipment Safety: It should also be emphasised that electrotherapy equipment should never be left unsupervised on any animal. I have seen many cases of applicators and equipment that have been damaged in the few moments left with the animal. This is particularly the case with horses being treated with pulsed magnetic therapy (PFMT). Normally phototherapy is a modality that requires the therapist to apply it throughout the treatment time. However, there are phototherapy applicators coming on the market that are flexible and may be strapped around limbs. The potential to suffer the same fate as PFMT applicators is possible if left even for very short periods.

Chapter Two

PHOTOTHERAPY APPLICATION AND DOSAGES

Niels Rydberg Finsen 1860 – 1904, a Danish physician, is credited as being the founder of modern phototherapy. He studied the effects of red light on living organisms and became aware of the antibacterial effects. The Finsen Institute in Copenhagen was first called the Finsen Medical Light Institute and was founded in 1896. Further study declined in favour of radiation therapy including ultraviolet that was developed in bacteriology research. However, serious up to date phototherapy, using the visible part of the electromagnetic spectrum and its fringes, began with the development of LASERs back in the early 1960s. Ruby lasers emitting visible red-light beams at 693nm were researched to see if any effect would be damaging to tissue if exposed to the high intensity beam. First experiments were used on shaven mice resulting in no negative effects and a surprisingly rapid regrowth of the hair compared with control groups. Thus began photo bio-stimulation studies, also referred to as bio-modulation, and the advent of phototherapy as we now understand it.

Figure 2. illustrates part of the electromagnetic spectrum radiated by the sun. The visible part of the spectrum ranges from around 400 to 700nm. Phototherapy, for the purposes of this book, extends well into the infrared. It is interesting to note that the peak output of the sun is around 470nm blue. This will be discussed when looking at specific effects of this wavelength and will be revisited for a more in-depth discussion later in the book.

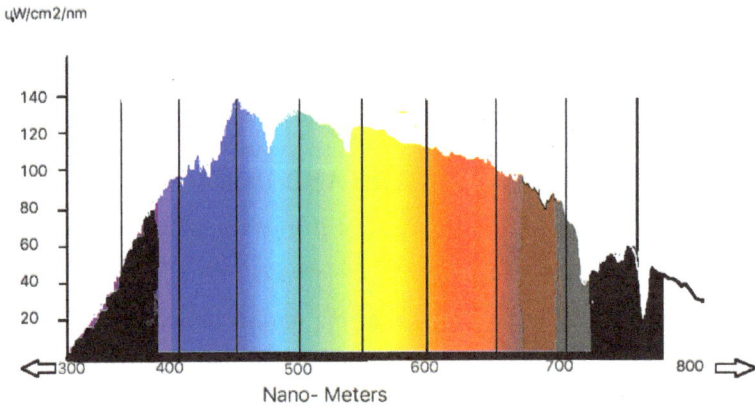

Figure 2. Spectral radiance output of the sun

It has long been known that moderate exposure to sunlight can be beneficial and that vitamin D synthesis in the skin is stimulated by ultraviolet light B category (UVB) - in fact over 90% is provided this way. But over exposure of UVA and UVB can destroy vitamin A, also known as retinol, and affect the immune system. Vitamin A is found in beta-carotene from vegetables. UVC can cause skin tumours if also over exposed. The differences between UVA, UVB and UVC are the frequency of the photons that light is made up of. This is directly related to the energy value of each photon and how it is absorbed into tissue. In the next chapter energy levels will be considered, but for this discussion, therapeutic phototherapy in the visible range is the main topic. Sunlight can be used in therapy as it is a mixture of all the colours and specific ones can reach different depths in tissue and have different effects. Light from the sun at ground level is generally a very pale yellow because part of the blue component is filtered by the atmosphere, resulting in a blue sky. However, treating specific injuries requires a knowledge of both the theory and application techniques that are largely dependent upon the type of injury to be treated and the frequency, ergo colour, being used.

A Guide to Phototherapy

My first introduction to the beneficial effects of light came when my younger son was born prematurely. He suffered from neonatal-natal jaundice and was placed in an incubator with a series of strip lights over him. His eyes were bound and after a short time he recovered and developed normally. The link between light and neonatal jaundice treatment intrigued me, especially how this treatment method came about. Under-developed livers in premature infants cannot process the bile pigment bilirubin and so it builds up in the blood stream, causing the skin to appear yellow. Exposure to light causes the molecular structure of bilirubin to change into a form (water soluble isomers) that can be processed by the infant's liver. Without treatment, a condition called Kernicterus can develop and may cause movement disorders and possibly mental disorders, as well as hearing loss in those children that survive. Phototherapy is now the standard treatment for neonatal jaundice. Strip lighting was used because it has a high content of ultraviolet radiation and it is this penetration of superficial veins that directly affects the bilirubin in the venal blood stream.

This discovery, according to the story of its use, came about when a laboratory sample of blood containing serum bilirubin was left for a short time on a windowsill, exposed to sunlight. When eventually it was tested it was found to be changed to the form that can be processed by infants. Blue light is now more commonly used in special incubators. Although very successful, it must be monitored very closely as there may be some side effects to over exposure. It is unlikely that direct risk from over exposure will occur when used in therapy, as timing is calculated to deliver specific doses to wounds and lesions and should not cause problems to underlying tissue, although eyes should always be protected. Over exposure to blue light can be the cause of retinal damage. This damage mainly occurs at the higher frequency end of the blue light spectrum. This will be further discussed in chapter eight when discussing research.

If injuries are superficial, as in lesions and bruises, then phototherapy may be a very useful modality using either blue or visible red applicators. Slightly deeper injuries, but still relatively superficial, can make use of longer wavelengths as with infrared radiation. In chapter six of this book we will investigate depths to which the primary sources of phototherapy can be effective at energy levels related to colour. In this early chapter, we need to discuss the therapy and the conditions and contraindications to it.

Categorising injuries falls into broad types arising from trauma. Kicks, head butts and sideswipes may not break skin but may damage underlying tissue. These can result in oedema, bruising and initially acute pain, becoming chronic, as healing begins to take place. Other injuries can arise from tumbles, stumbles, burns and skeletal injuries producing the same reactions as above but also open injuries. In addition, other problems such as skin conditions including dermatitis, eczema, erythema nodosum and other forms may be encountered. Using phototherapy to help resolve some of these issues depends upon location and accessibility. Accessibility would apply both to where the injury is located on the animal and to where it is possible to apply therapy, i.e. in a field, stable, kennels or even in the owner's home.

So, before any treatment commences a risk assessment needs to be carried out to determine any underlying problems that could affect the therapy following a set regime. For the professional therapist, there needs to be a report from a veterinary surgeon who will diagnose the condition. Only veterinary surgeons are qualified to diagnose and the therapist, based upon this diagnosis, will follow up by determining a course of suitable treatment to aid recovery. So, armed with a veterinary diagnosis and referral of the injury, the therapist determines the electrotherapy to be used and, for our purposes, that one is phototherapy.

The most obvious injuries ideally suited to phototherapy are those causing lesions. These can be rips, tears and those arising from surgical procedures. They can also include scratches and scrapes, in fact any type that may open tissue to the environment and cause bleeding. Following surgical procedures, it is likely that a dressing covers the wound on small animals for an initial period but with larger ones, depending upon location, they are often stitched and, as with tears, left mostly uncovered. In this situation exposure to bacteria could be a problem and in the early stages mitigating the problem may be helped by using blue phototherapy. It has been well established that shorter wavelengths such as blue and ultraviolet, as studied by Finsen, have an antibacterial affect. The possible mechanisms of how this is effective is discussed in chapter six.

Depending upon the applicator, the dimensions of the wound should be noted and treated on a point by point basis. Most surgical wounds are long and provide a definable line of injury. Treatment times are currently based upon minimum energy calculations of 1 joule/cm^2 although some sources recommend up to 3 joules/cm^2 (Baxter). **Light intensities vary with the** type of light source used, also with pulsating frequency. When pulsed, the percentage ratio between on and off times needs to be noted but it does not necessarily affect timing as other underlying effects may be taking place that may increase its efficacy. Pulsing light is also believed to increase therapeutic effectiveness as it allows an assimilation time for cells to process the changes caused by the absorption of photons and reduce the opacity of tissue.

To calculate dosage:

Remember 1 joule per second = 1 Watt. If power available is 5mW/cm^2 or 5/1000 Watts/cm^2, reciprocating this by dividing the 5 into 1000 will give the time in seconds per joule transferred under perfect conditions.

1000/5 = 200 seconds to transfer 1 joule/cm^2

It is essential to know the joules/cm^2 from any device. If an overall power rating is given, say 80mW from a cluster, divide this by the active area of the emitters in cm^2.

Example: 80mW = total output. Active emitter area = 6cm^2.

Output per cm^2 = 80/6mW/cm^2 = 13.3mW/cm^2.

Divide this into 1000: 1000/13.3 = 75 seconds

So, the time needed to transfer 1 joule per each cm^2 = 75 seconds.

For each 6cm^2 of active head area, 6 joules in total would be transferred. If this is regarded as a 'point', then the area to be treated in cm^2 would need to be divided by 6 if greater than the head area. Each 'point' would require 75 seconds until all area divisions of 6cm^2 have been covered for each session.

Remember these calculations are based on the ideal conditions providing direct access to tissue. In real life, colour of skin and hair thickness get in the way of direct access and affect energy transfer. Adjustments to timing would have to be increased, especially if 2 or 3 j/cm^2 is desired. Higher powered applicators would use the same calculating method. Using a true laser, as with a cluster applicator with an embedded laser(s), may slightly confuse the calculations but if the manufacturers have stated an overall power rating for the head then measure the active area (point) and use that in the calculations. The embedded lasers would only cover a small area but would be overlapped by the emitter cluster. A single true laser pen may have the power rating given as the spot power or milli-Watts/cm^2 (mW/cm^2).

Most experienced therapists usually develop a set routine that works for them for the variety of conditions presented. Calculations and the table below should serve to act as a guide and are for perfect conditions.

A Guide to Phototherapy

Emitter rated output in milli-Watts	Time to deliver 1 joule/cm² (seconds)	Emitter rated output in milli-Watts	Time to deliver 1 joule/cm2 (seconds)
0.5	2000	10	100
1.0	1000	20	50
2.0	500	30	33
3.0	333	50	20
4.0	250	100	10
5.0	200	200	5.0
7.0	143	500	2.0

Table 1. Energy transfer timings for a single emitter covering 1cm².

Treatment Methods:

These depend upon applicator types, either a pen type or cluster. For each type, the area covered by the light beam is called a 'point', as mentioned above. The size of the point depends on the number of emitters in the applicator and the active area being directly applied to the target area. If we set the treatment area as 1cm² as a reference and a minimum, then a pen held close to the lesion would require a time dependent upon the stated power per point (in this case 1cm²). Using a blue or red pen rated at 5mW output would require 200 seconds to deliver just one joule. This may seem a long process for a wound of length 10cm and greater, however using a cluster would substantially reduce this. Also, other factors come into play dependent upon frequency. The primary function of using blue light along the length of a wound is to stop bacterial proliferation and invasion into the lesion. Blue is quickly dispersed, both into the first couple of mm and laterally from the head. This would simply mean that a point of treatment may be at greater distances than the 1cm² intervals due to dispersion overlap. It also means that the amount of energy required to stop or kill the bacteria could be additive between the treatment points, as research has shown that a lateral effect from the point of treatment is known to occur. This will be discussed later.

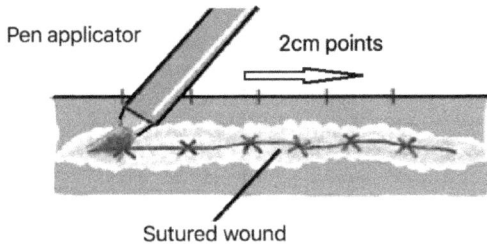

Pen applicator   2cm points

Sutured wound

Figure 3. Treatment points along a sutured wound

This indicates that the most effective part of the beam is central to the emitter at the surface. However, an overlapping treatment at short intervals between each point would radiate each side of the emitter and effectively double the time exposure for those areas where the photon density is reduced. Table 1 provides a timing for minimum energy transfers under ideal conditions.

The above-mentioned table is for transferring 1 joule/cm^2 to skin surface under perfect conditions as previously stated. Timing for higher joules of energy is simply joules required multiplied by the time in seconds, as given above. The above table does not consider the effect of overlapping points or pulsing the beam. Pulsing the beam on a '50% on 50% off' basis may not affect the timing to any great extent. It may affect the depth that it reaches into tissue. This aspect that makes up for the 'off' time will be discussed later in chapter six and the frequency of the pulses will be discussed in the research chapter eight. The settings generally recommended are 1400Hz or, if not available, 200Hz and 50Hz. However, for some treatments others have suggested 100Hz to stimulate certain aspects of cells and this setting will be discussed in chapter eight.

Red light phototherapy may stimulate epithelial cell growth and reduce scarring. Providing that the wound is uninfected, this should be applied using a point by point application based on the above timings. If the wound shows any sign of being infected with an exudate such as pus leaking out, then, after treating over the full wound with blue light, red light should be followed but avoiding stimulating an area over the exudate fissure, so leaving an opening for drainage until the wound seals naturally. Pen type applicators treating a long thin wound on a point by point basis may be somewhat liberally applied in judging the closeness of each point. Red light disperses sub-dermally from the point of application and there has been some evidence of a photo-chemical effect extending laterally to this point. This is sometimes referred to as a series of specific biochemical reactions, as alluded to in the previous text. This is also discussed in later chapters

To summarize, blue light can be applied all over a wound including any exudate opening. Red light can be similarly applied over all the injury when the wound is sealed, but in early wounds avoids the point of where the exudate is leaking.

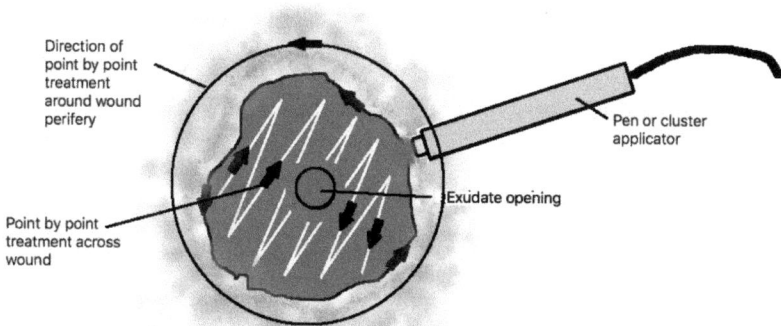

Figure 4. Applicator treatment around an open wound

Clusters are very useful to deliver treatment over a larger area. Treatment of any wound left open should follow the same principles as for narrow sutures. With this sort of injury, it will matter little that the treatment to the wound is only being applied from part of the cluster. Treat the cluster as a point and apply along the length of the wound. The same rules should apply to infected wounds and if a large area with a central exudate, then as in the previous paragraph, treat the whole wound except over the exudate area. This treatment would be continued, if possible, on a regular basis. This would ideally be daily with at least two treatments separated by a minimum of 4 hours. This is a standard timing from research for other forms of electrotherapies that allow biochemical reactions to be restored to their previous levels after treatment.

Deep wounds and damage to tissue may be best treated using other modalities that can penetrate further and are matched to the type of injury presented. Typical of these are pulsed magnetic therapy for orthopaedic injuries and deep soft tissue and swelling problems. Ultrasound (Shortwave) therapy, although penetrating deeper than phototherapy, suffers from rapid attenuation within a couple of cm. The lower frequency (long wave) has a greater depth penetration but carries proportionately less energy. If a superficial subdermal injury that has not broken skin is presented for treatment, phototherapy is the ideal modality using visible red applicators. It would take many volumes to list each type of injury suitable for treatment so generalisation is necessary to keep to the most common.

A hard knock or a collision will usually produce three probable responses in soft tissue: swelling, bruising and pain. Applying visible red phototherapy is the most appropriate for the superficial aspects of the injury. However, direct access to the affected area may be a problem. In the early stages of the injury palpation may be difficult due to sensitivity and may elicit a vocal or snapping response from a dog. Equine patients are possibly easier, but having direct access to skin may prove a problem due to the thickness of the hair. Of course, the same would also apply to any small furry animal.

Sometimes it may help to dampen the area with water. The effect of this may cause hairs to stick together, allowing some but limited access to the skin surface. Black or very dark hair will absorb red light, converting it into heat, although likely to be minimal and of   little, if any, therapeutic value. Dosage calculations would have to be extended to transfer therapeutic levels in cases where there is minimal skin exposure. Shaving the affected area may be another option, if the animal permits. Clusters may be useful over the injury area covered by hair, as some will filter down to the surface, but again calculating just how much of the light is at therapeutic levels is difficult. It may be that the hair itself acts as a conduit by transduction of visible red photons into infrared wavelengths.

Where irritation due to certain forms of bacteria is found around hair follicles, blue light pen application over the areas of irritation may alleviate the problem, but again accessing the affected area may need some prior planning. Pen applicators may be useful as they can be more easily pushed down to the skin surface amongst the hairs but really come into their own for injuries in hard to access areas such as under armpits and in other areas such as between toes. With all types of applicator, the need for hygiene is paramount due to the possibility of transferring pathogens between animals. Simply covering with sandwich 'cling' film pulled tightly over the active area of cluster or end of a pen to seal it and then hygienically discard after each treatment.

This chapter should be viewed as a general guide to the application of phototherapy as a modality of choice or as adjunct to the more physical techniques used in veterinary or human physiotherapy. The following table is a simple guide to what, and where, it is recommended for use. The timing of treatments to deliver a minimum dosage have not been included because, as stated in the text calculations, these are based on the ideal delivery of energy into tissue. In physics, this is referred to as 'black body' absorption where, in a perfect scenario, all (100%) of the radiant energy is absorbed without any reflections. Clearly in the real world this is not the case, therefore practitioners will develop their own timing techniques based on the conditions encountered when patients are referred and responses noted.

Injury Type	Suitability	Pen	Cluster	Infrared
Open wound	Yes	Red and blue	Red	No
Sutured wound	Yes	Blue	Red	No
Infected wound	No	Blue	Blue	No
Non-infected wound	No	Red	Red	No
Bruising and swelling	Yes	Red	Red	Possibly, if deep injury
Muscle tears	Yes, if superficially presented	Red	Red	Yes
Tendon injuries	Yes, if superficially accessible	Red	Red	Yes
Surface scar tissue	Yes	Red	Red	No
Subcutaneous scar tissue	Yes	Red	Red	Yes
Ulcers	Yes	Blue	No	No
Tumours	Yes, under veterinary supervision	Blue/ Red	Blue/ Red	No
Blemishes and burns	As for tumours	Red	Red	No
Acne	Yes	Blue	Blue	No

Table 2. Recommended treatments for a variety of injuries

The above table is for guidance only as empirical research is limited for most of the above; anecdotal evidence suggests positive outcomes in these areas. Although the above table shows little recommendation for infrared it should not be excluded, but ideally kept for deeper injuries. The use of this range of light frequencies from 880 to 950nm is popular and anecdotally effective. Higher powered infrared class IV 800nm infrared devices may be utilised for many conditions but extreme care must be taken for both patient, practitioner and owner/observer.

Before concluding this chapter, the use of phototherapy as an acupuncture point stimulator needs consideration. Acupuncture, in its purest form, is the puncturing of the skin at specific locations to derive certain effects. It is frequently regarded as pseudoscience in the explanations of its mechanisms. Arising from Chinese traditional medicine it has found a place in alternative medical practice in the west. Acupuncture points are located at certain meridian points around the body located on the skin surface. These are said to be stimulated by penetrating them with fine needles and have individual significance to various organs within the body. There is no scientific evidence that these meridian lines exist and in Chinese medicine are described as 'lines of energy flow', again not verified by scientific investigation. However, some benefits have been shown to be effective. Becker's research (1985) into the existence of 'peri-neural currents' may offer an insight as to what exactly acupuncture points are.

Peri-neural currents arise from charges at the brain stem, possibly caused by the fact that the two hemispheres of the brain are un-balanced in terms of volume, and the orientation of neurons in each side electrically oppose each other. This orientation is proven by direct induction into the brain of electric charges by trans-cranial stimulation. Research at Sheffield University found that the polarity of the electromagnetic pulses affects the polarity of charges differently in each hemisphere, causing action potentials to be initiated and detected by efferent reactions throughout the body. This difference in orientation between the two cranial hemispheres may lead to a slight imbalance of overall electric charge arising from neuronal cellular orientation and cellular charges. Minute electric currents would naturally flow between the hemispheres both locally and measurably throughout the body caused by these small potential differences, manifesting as a polarised charge between left and right sides. Also, Carlos Matteucci (1811- 1868 and Du Bois-Reymond (1818-1896)... both known for their work identifying cellular voltages and action potentials, postulated about and then measured current flow across lesions. Du Bois-Reymond found these currents to be in the order of one micro-amp. These detectable currents may flow more easily and be distributed around the body through glial cell cytosol.

Becker verified the existence of such minute current flows using 'Hall effect' experiments. Peri-neural currents is the term applied to them. It was suggested that parts of glial cells would allow cell to cell contact where each myelin segment makes some physical contact with the adjacent ones. Current then flows more easily through micro-apertures between each contact point. This allows micro-currents to flow along the length of the nerve and its branches, completing millions of circuits loops back to the brain.

Electrical conductivity measured between two points at certain locations appears to be very much raised at places commonly used as acupuncture points. It is possible that nerve bunching or small neural ganglions at these points cause these changes in conductivity. Stimulating with fine needles would have a cause and effect on areas of the body from locations served by those nerves by both directly interfering with them, and by also affecting micro current flows in that area. As far as the veterinary therapist is concerned in the UK, only specifically trained veterinary surgeons can apply acupuncture using needles to animal patients. Therapists use non-invasive techniques such as phototherapy to try to achieve some effect.

In later chapters, the discussion into how photons affect general biological structures will be covered. However, at this point it is sufficient to state that the effect from cyclooxygenase in cell cytosol being stimulated by photons is the release of nitric oxide and inhibition of prostaglandins. The release of nitric oxide causes localised vasodilation. Inhibition of prostaglandin production reduces pain sensations. It is these that may have some positive effects on both nerve signal transmission and peri-neural current flow at these acupuncture points. Research, now, is both lacking and inconsistent regarding beneficial effects. This has resulted in most reports being anecdotal. No guidance can be given on the timing but if any effect is to be achieved, then red light phototherapy should be the main colour used.

This chapter has so far laid the foundations for the understanding and basic treatment regime for phototherapy. Dose calculations and application times provide values that depend upon many factors and conditions. Many practitioners use phototherapy pens to stimulate acupuncture points and treat around trigger points. Most of the reported success in these areas are verbal or documented as case reports. Research is difficult to prove anecdotes but often there is an overwhelming case to accept at face value based on large amounts of feedback.

Contraindications to some types of phototherapy are relatively few, however some antibiotics can cause problems, particularly when exposed to UVA light. This frequency is just above the high end of the deep visible blue spectrum. Because animals in most cases are fully covered by hair, direct exposure to sunlight is blocked by this, therefore it may not present such a large problem, except on short haired breeds of dogs. However, precautions should always be taken if the veterinary surgeon prescribes any of the most common tetracyclines such as tetracycline itself and doxycycline, as they are known to induce photo-toxic reactions. The full list is extensive and even includes anti-inflammatory drugs, such as ibuprofen. The higher the colour frequency the more toxic the effect.

An important factor in applying phototherapy is that it does not require a coupling agent as is the case with ultrasound therapy. Efficacy may be increased by dampening fur to allow access to skin surfaces but never use a gel or oil-based cream. This could become very hot and may cause heat burns in a relatively short time. The ideal is a dry and matt surface over the area to be treated, so if dampening is used, keep it limited. This also avoids harmful reflections of wet and shiny target areas, although in any case, eye protection should be worn.

The next chapter of the book starts to visit the whys and wherefores of this modality and to take the reader into a study of relationships between light, photons, wavelengths and colours. It will be necessary to visit the basics of physics and a little chemistry to achieve an understanding of this.

Chapter Three

THE SCIENCE UNDERPINNING LIGHT PRODUCTION

All life has evolved in a radiation rich environment. Most of this radiation goes unnoticed except for where we can physically detect it through our senses or through dedicated equipment such as radios, TVs, Geiger counters etc. We ourselves generate and radiate photons in the far infrared range as well as absorbing and reflecting photons in other ranges. At any one time, millions of radiative particles pass through every one of us, from outer space, in the form of cosmic radiation. It could be postulated that our evolution has possibly been shaped by radiation, allowing the survival of species resistant to its negative effects. Human and animal senses detect radiation from within a very narrow band of the extremely wide spectrum.

Whilst some radiation is in the form of particles emanating from decay of atoms, as with alpha and beta radiation, positrons etc, virtually all others are electromagnetic in the form of 'photons' that have both a frequency and an energy component. Radio frequency transmissions, as with radio, television and radar etc., share a common speed of transmission with photons but are derived directly from electron flows. Photons come directly from within atoms themselves. Humans and animals have evolved systems that effectively are 'tuned' to certain frequencies and the most obvious of these are contained within and around the visible part of the spectrum as specialised cells in the eyes. Phototherapy makes use of specific frequencies of light, to either enhance that which is naturally received or so that we can make use of in assisting the healing process where tissue is damaged. It is necessary to understand the basics of photon generation and energy levels within atoms to appreciate that there is a direct link between them. Where electrons are, through external stimulation, caused to jump to a higher energy level, the 'excited' electron then returns to its original level and in doing so releases the initial stimulative energy as an electro-magnetic particle, the photon. The energy carried by the photon then equals the difference between the two-energy level exchanges and has a frequency component.

Light forms a small part of the electromagnetic spectrum. It has very high frequencies such that it is normal to state wavelengths of light rather than actual frequency. The ultimate speed is said to be that at which light travels and is given as around 300,000,000, specifically 299,792,458 meters per second. The wave length of a frequency is given in nano-meters (nm) that is thousand millionth of a meter, so, taking a wavelength within the red part of the visible spectrum around 630nm, that means 630 nano-meters wave lengths would be passing a point in space at the speed of light. This would give a frequency of:

(1000,000,000/630 x 299,792,458) Hz or 475861044444444.4Hz, simplified as 476THz.

At this high frequency range, all light radiation is easily reflected or absorbed by solid objects depending upon colours from across the spectrum. White objects reflect almost all frequencies whereas black absorption is the opposite, absorbing almost all. Some of that reflected light ends up being focussed in the eyes to give visible perception of the world around, based upon the intensity of reflections and absorption of materials that can be solid, liquid or gaseous objects. Some materials absorb visible light dependant on colour or allow its passage through it almost unimpeded, such as glass. However, animal and human tissue can have varying degrees of absorption and translucency, absorbing from ultra violet to visible and infrared light within certain limits. Understanding how light is generated is therefore fundamental to understanding phototherapy. The early part of this book will look at the science aspects and reflects on it as the book progresses through the subject.

For the reader with little or no scientific background then the next few paragraphs may help refresh understanding of the structure of the atoms and molecules. The bonding and sharing of electrons by various atoms provides a background in learning about molecular structure and how bonds may be broken by various energetic means, from physical mechanical collisions with objects, to extraneous electrons or photons making contact at light speed with individual atoms. The latter is the form of stimulation which is implemented in phototherapy, both in photon production and in tissue stimulation. Natural stimulation is all around and the result of these 'collisions' leads to a release of photons, both within the visible part of the electromagnetic spectrum and beyond either extremities as part of the invisible spectrum.

Certain types of quartz easily give out a flash of light when physically struck with a hard object. The energy from the blow displaces some electrons from within the atomic structure, effectively storing some of that energy, but only momentarily. As the electrons recombine with the atoms, the stored energy is released as photons of visible light. This is a visible example of the piezo-electric effect that exists all around in nature and is made use of by the body as part of the maintenance of bones. In bone, the piezo-electric effect is from hydroxyapatite that has similar crystalline structures to those found in silicon. Silicon forms the basis of most modern electronic devices, especially in light generation. By specially treating the silicon, light can be generated continuously and then used in therapy. This will be covered in depth later, but first the refresher on atomic structure and electron exchanges within them.

The three main components common to all matter are electrons, protons and neutrons. In atoms, the balance in numbers of electrons to protons maintains an electrical neutrality. The number of electrons orbiting a nucleus, which is made up of protons and neutrons, should also equal the number of protons within that nucleus. For simplicity atoms are usually illustrated as below, see Fig 5, with electrons 'orbiting' at varying energy levels around the nucleus. The study of quantum physics looks at the arrangement and the energy of electrons within the atom along with the influences that can release 'quanta' amounts of energy, hereon referred to as photons.

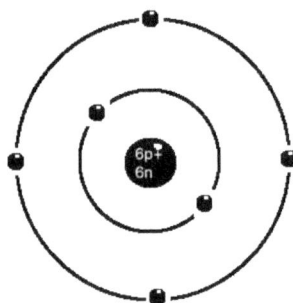

Figure 5. Typical illustration of a carbon atom

The above illustration is typical to show the formation of a carbon atom. The nucleus contains six protons and six neutrons. The six electrons orbit at different energy levels, also known as 'clouds' or shells. Electrons are very much smaller than the illustration suggests but for clarity they are shown larger. The electrons are highly energetic and orbit the nucleus forming a cloud, such that at the level closest to the nucleus (known as ground state level) there is a maximum of two electrons at this level and in other larger atoms this level holds the same number. Electrons have a negative charge and, as like charges repel, it is this repulsion that limits the maximum to two electrons within the confines and sub levels of the cloud at this first level.

At the second level, where just four electrons form the cloud in the carbon atom, the area the cloud covers is geometrically larger and could, in fact, hold up to eight electrons in the level. If a level or shell is filled to its maximum capacity then it becomes very stable. Since carbon has only 4 electrons in its second level it can achieve maximum stability by borrowing and sharing electrons from neighbouring atoms such as oxygen. Oxygen normally exists as O_2. By sharing electrons, each atom effectively fills its outer shell with 8 electrons, even though only six exist in the outer shell of singlet oxygen. This then becomes an oxygen molecule:

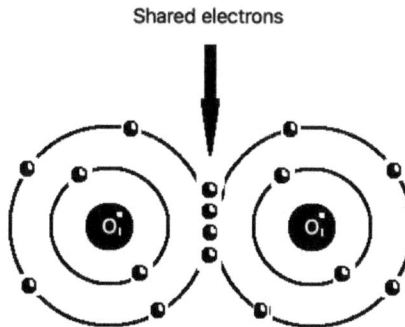

Figure 6. Oxygen molecule

High amounts of energy can cause singlet oxygen to join with carbon to form carbon monoxide. The carbon effectively 'borrows' 4 of the oxygen's six electrons to make up the eight required to give a more stable outer shell whilst the oxygen borrows two from the carbon to make up the eight in its own outer shell. Similarly, CO_2 utilises two electrons from each oxygen outer shell to make up its own eight whilst each oxygen atom shares two electrons from the carbon atom to each make up its own eight outer shell formations.

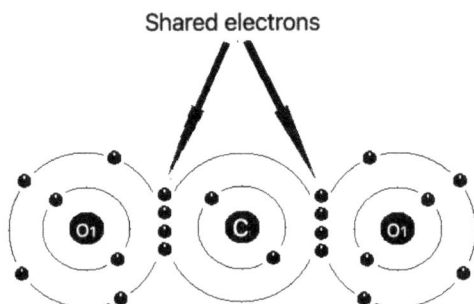

Figure 7. Carbon dioxide molecule.

The above concept is not difficult to comprehend if, from a point of view of one of the oxygen atoms, it 'sees' two of the electrons from the carbon to make up its eight whilst the other oxygen atom 'sees' and shares the other two. The carbon atom co-sharing two electrons from each oxygen atom has effectively filled its outer shell to its stable maximum. This sort of bonding of molecular structures is called co-valent bonding and the outer shell or cloud is called the valence shell.

Understanding the basics of molecular structures is also fundamental to understanding energy exchanges within these sorts of structures or from within individual atoms. It should be noted that in the above, and in similar structures making up different molecules, electrons are so energetic that all the valence electrons would be sharing and orbiting all the atoms maintaining both stability and electrical balance. But starting from the simplest atom, hydrogen, we can see how electrons orbit forming the cloud or shell but have different levels or sub shells formed by electrons but still obeying the rules of maximums per shell: 2, 8, 18, 32, 50.... per each energy level respectively. The key to understanding how light is generated is to investigate how electrons can not only form the basis of an electric current, and subsequently form magnetic fields, but how they can change position between energy levels and sub levels through external influences. These forced changes in levels cause the release of packets of electromagnetic energy, known as photons, as the electrons regain their original positions, returning to their original energy state.

Depending on the level of experience with physics and chemistry, it is ideal to understand energy levels and sub levels to begin to further understand how different wavelengths of light can be generated from exchanges of electrons between these levels and sub levels. Taking the simplest atom, hydrogen, in its singlet form, it will have only one level and one sub level where the single electron orbits in the cloud it forms. This is called the orbital and can be given a designator letter 's' so hydrogen has $1s^1$. 's' orbitals are always spherical but in larger atoms more complex orbitals labelled 'p', 'd' and 'f' have more complex shapes, but still follow the rule of maximums for the number of electrons within that shell or energy level. If we take carbon, that has a configuration of 2 electrons in the first shell and sub-shell and four at the next energy level, then it can be given a sub-shell configuration of $1s^2$, $2p^2$ $2d^2$.

A general order of shells and sub shells follows: 1s 2s 2p 3s 3p 4s 3d 4p 5s 4d 5p 6s 4f 5d 6p 7s 5f 6d 7p. The number is the level position with 1 starting at ground state. The superscripted number usually attached to a specific level will show the number of electrons within the level and sub-level that will never exceed the maximum for that level following the order 2, 8, 18, 32, 50, 72. The orbitals for p, d and f sub-levels can be in x, y and z planes and can be shown as an angular figure of 8 shape. In the diagram below just one shape is shown.

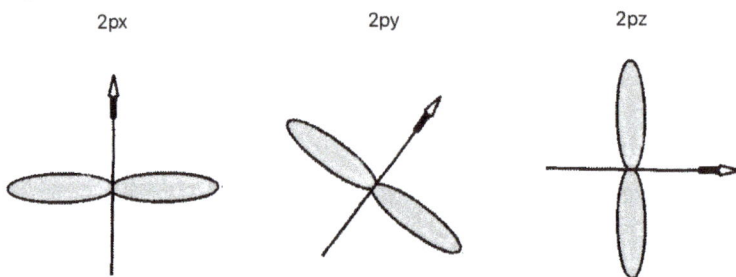

Figure 8. Sub-level orbitals.

The above shows orbits for sub-levels $2p_x$, $2p_y$ and $2p_z$. 2s would always be a spherical shape. Electrons form the X, Y and Z three dimensional shapes. Although the subject may seem complex to the non-physicist it allows a more logical understanding of how different molecules bond and their shapes form by the sharing of electrons from within sub-levels. However, for the purposes of this book our interest is in the generation of light from within atoms due to electrons being displaced by external energetic forces momentarily storing energy and then releasing it as the electron is returned to its correct level or sub-level.

All radiant energy is electromagnetic and can occupy any position within the electromagnetic spectrum. Detectors of this radiation are matched physically to specific radiation frequencies or optimised within a 'bandwidth' of such frequencies. Very low frequency electronically generated electromagnetic waves are used to send messages around the world since they will follow the curvature of the earth. As the frequency increases electromagnetic energy becomes more directional, largely following a line of sight transmission. At frequencies from 20Khz to several hundred kilo-hertz, they can still penetrate solid structures such as buildings etc., and follow the earth's curvature, and are known as HF (high frequencies).

As frequencies increase, this earth curvature-following and building-penetration ability becomes very much reduced. Very High Frequency (VHF) and Ultra High Frequency (UHF) ranges generally follow a straight line of sight transmission. As frequencies increase to beyond those used in radio transmissions, radiation comes straight from within atomic structures. What we perceive visually of the world around us is from a very narrow band of the electromagnetic spectrum, visible light. Common to all these examples is the speed of transmission, light speed. Phototherapy is generally concentrated on the visible parts of the spectrum, (see Fig 9.) and its fringes as part of the invisible ultraviolet and infrared ends.

This energy, and that from around the visible fringes, directly influences biological tissue and may be largely beneficial. The effect on tissue is frequency dependant as different energy levels are a function of frequency affecting its ability to penetrate the skin's surface.

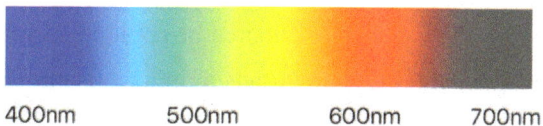

400nm   500nm   600nm   700nm

Figure 9. Visible part of the electromagnetic spectrum given in nano-metres (nm). Actual photograph taken from direct sunlight through a prism by the author.

The frequencies involved are produced by electrons changing energy levels within the atomic levels and sub-level orbitals, and are themselves a function of the amount of energy released from this. Energy emitted directly from within atomic structures as a photon is of a pure frequency. Human eyes perceive colour by having an overlapping sensitivity to three specific primary colours, red, green and blue. A mixture of these colours gives virtually all others by being processed by the optical cortex of the brain. Red, green and blue are known as the primary colours in light. The three specifically combined give a perception of white. However, a green optical filter will block red light and yellow will block blue. Conversely a blue filter will block yellow light and a red filter will block green light. Each filter absorbs photons of a specific colour in its own atomic structure, that is then either agitated, causing an increase in temperature, or re-emitted at a different non-visible frequency. In either case it obeys the laws on conservation of energy. Modern flat screen televisions and monitors utilise a LCD matrix in triads of red, green and blue to form the liquid crystal pixels. By varying each colour density, all colours of the spectrum can be made as the backlight passes through them. Whilst the bright backlight provides all the frequencies of colour as a bright white light source, the liquid crystals making up the pixels absorb all other colours, with individual ones in each triad allowing just one of the primary colours to pass through it. The cleverly designed electronics determines just how much of each colour is allow through, with millions of them making up the colour image. Large screen public display boards use three different coloured bright light sources, usually light emitting diodes (LEDs), arranged in triads forming the large display matrix.

Television cameras and digital cameras sometimes utilise a prism system to divide the image into three colours through red, green and blue filters. Electronic charged couple devices (ccd) capture these images and process them before recombining them into an electronic image captured in full colour. The ccd receptor is a matrix of light sensitive components that convert the image into electrical signals. This is similar, but on a very much smaller and less complex scale, than the human eye perceives colour. These photo receptor cells are discussed in chapter eight. Theories that have a common base between the absorption and processing of colour within the eye will also be put forward as to how such colours are absorbed into and affect tissue.

Chapter Four

PHOTONS: THE ENIGMATIC ENTITY.

Photons are an energy form that make up nearly all the electromagnetic spectrum and come directly from within the structure of atoms. They are enigmatic in that they exhibit different qualities of being both a particle and a wave. The wave is effectively the frequency component exhibited by photons but the particle aspect acts individually and carries a specific amount of energy. It is not the purpose of this book to deeply involve the reader in quantum physics, but brushing alongside the subject helps to give an understanding of the transduction of photons as energy packages into other forms that are beneficial when directed as a therapy. Phototherapy takes its name from the photon, as does photography. This name was coined from Einstein's photo electric paper by Gilbert N. Lewis, who used the term photon in a letter to the editor of Nature Magazine in 1926. The term photon was used to describe a quantum of energy that had the characteristics of a wave but also that of a particle. In the case of therapy, perhaps a better name for its therapeutic use would be 'photon-therapy', so phototherapy can be viewed as a slight contraction of a more appropriate title.

Max Planck (1858 – 1947) gave his name to Planck's constant - this provides a value for the energy in an individual photon. This energy is directly related to the frequency of the photon. Blue light has around twice the energy per photon that infrared has, i.e. infrared at 950nm has exactly half the energy of blue at 475nm. Planck's research gave a precise value of:

$6.626070040(81) \times 10^{-34}\,\text{J}^{-1}$ as a constant.

Multiplying this constant by the frequency gives the value in joules per photon and is given the symbol 'h'. Actual frequency is given the Greek symbol 'v' so E (energy in joules) = hv. If we take our example from the previous chapter of visible red light at 630nm wavelength, the frequency was around 476.2 x 10^{12}Hz. Multiplying this by Planck's constant gives a good approximation of:

$6.626 \times 10^{-34} \times 476.2 \times 10^{12} = 3.155 \times 10^{-19}$ joules per photon.

This energy is the same as the amount absorbed by an electron by initial stimulation, causing it to change its energy state to higher levels within atoms. Put simply, an electron forced into a higher energy state by whatever stimulation, say from E_1 to E_2, then the energy released as a photon is calculated as follows:

E_{photon} = Frequency x Planck's constant (hv).

So, $hv = E_2 - E_1$

Stimulus

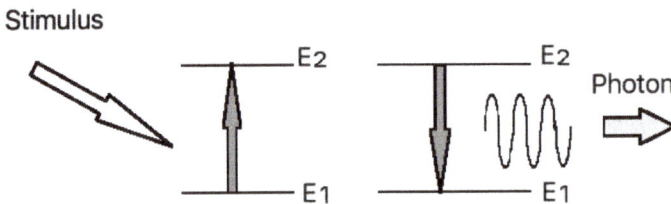

Figure 10. Simplified view of electron stimulation and energy release

For the therapist, these figures are just an exercise to gain a deeper understanding of energy transfers and the therapeutic levels of transfers of energy will be discussed later in the book. However, it may be of interest to show an approximation of the massive volume of photons required to transfer a single joule of energy by simply inverting the above value:

i.e. $1 / 3.155 \times 10^{-19} = 3.17 \times 10^{18}$ photons, which is about the equivalent to just under value of half the number of average size grains of sand on all the beaches of the earth.

A Guide to Phototherapy

How photons are generated and gain this energy comes back to energy levels in atoms, as previously discussed, and the energetic properties of electrons. The connection between electrons and electromagnetism is well established when they are caused to leave their atoms. They effectively leap from atom to atom in an orderly direction as they 'drift' along a conducting wire or within the molecular structures of certain metals. This movement of electrons generates a magnetic field at right angles to the flow. When contained within atoms, electrons exchange places within their atoms due to stimulation from external sources. As they gain energy they jump to a higher energy level or sub-level. Electrons within that original energy level effectively gain energy from the stimulus, this being either from another electron collision or another photon. This electron, crossing to a higher energy level, exceeds the maximum for that level and is then caused to jump back to its pre-stimulus original level. The energy stored is then released as a photon and the amount of energy depends upon how much was originally used to displace it to the higher energy level. This difference in the amount of electromagnetic energy is proportionated to the frequency and is the difference in energy between the two levels. See Fig 10. above.

The amount of energy in a photon can be extremely high, as with gamma and X-rays. These can be useful in medical diagnostics and some treatments, provided exposure time is limited. They have the same properties in terms of speed of transmission but, being of a very high frequency, carry proportionately high amounts of energy that can be damaging to biological tissue if over exposed.

One aspect that has been little discussed or researched is the amplitude of the photon and its duration. This may be purely academic, but if a higher energy electron is returned across several energy levels then the energy released would be $E_n - O_{riginal}$, where E_n is the energy level to which the electron is stimulated to, and $E_{original}$ its original pre-stimulus level. It can be assumed that as the electrons are accelerated back to the original level, the emitted radiation starts as soon as transit starts. The high speed of electron transit depends on the amount of energy causing the electron's displacement. Returning to its original level releases this energy. Higher energy released due to the higher charge would cause a sharp rate of the release of the radiation, hence the higher frequency, and a larger amplitude in comparison to lower energy transits. It is also probable that the single slope illustrating the rate of release of radiation emitted would form a damped oscillation per photon.

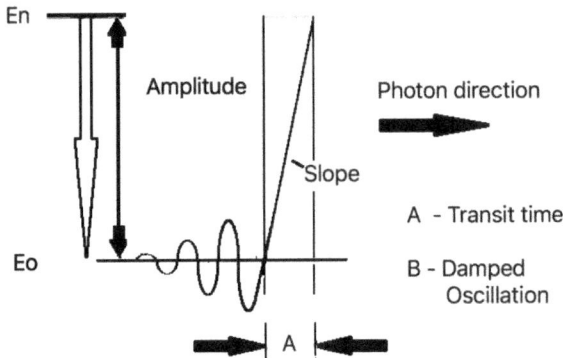

Figure 11. A theory of photon emission process.

The above diagram (Fig. 11.) is a simplified *possible* theoretical view of the emission process. The emission of photonic energy from the electron transit starts as a wave-front emitted throughout the transit time 'A' as the electron transits back from En to Eo, Eo 'o' in this case being the energy level of origin, not necessarily ground state. In real terms, the transit time 'A' equals the reciprocal of the frequency or the time of one full wavelength. Taking visible red frequency of 475861044444444.4 Hz, then reciprocating this gives a transit time of 2.1×10^{-15} seconds. The radiated wave then falls off to the Eo, the original energy level or balanced state, as the photon energy is released at light speed in the direction of the arrow. This also shows a trailing damped oscillation caused by the momentum of the electron settling back in the level and forming the basis of the photon's frequency

Summarising this model: the initial energy release slope and trailing damped oscillation provides the frequency of the photon and the distance between En to Eo the amplitude. Using the above: Planck's constant x (1/$\delta y/\delta A$)$\approx$(hv) = En – Eo where $\delta y/\delta A$ is the slope derived from A, δA is the transit time and δy the change in amplitude. A would also correspond to the wavelength of the photon, equating to the time from peak to peak of a single wave. A damped oscillation would follow mathematically where $\delta y/\delta t$ sin(x) = 0. This corresponds to the maximum rate change and may be formed from the inertia of the electron slightly overrunning the original (Eo) level on return. It would then eventually return to zero. If the distance transited by the electron is shorter due to less energetic initial stimulation, then the energy release slope would be less steep and δA longer, hence the frequency component and energy component less. This discussion is my own theory but may fit in with the facts of higher frequency (steeper release slope) and amplitude providing the photon with an amount of energy proportionate to both frequency and amplitude.

Representation of the energy bands in which electrons naturally reside forming clouds can be seen in the following diagram, (Fig. 12). This is a standardised method of representing electrons externally stimulated to move to higher energy levels emitting energy when returning to their original levels. The ionisation level is that level where electrons are energised to totally leave the atom.

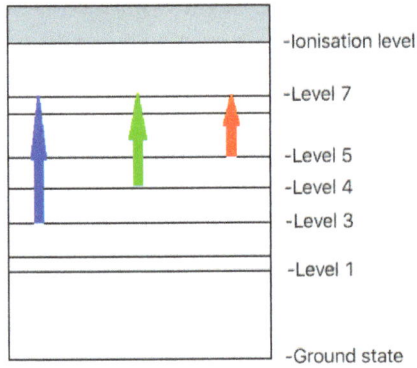

Figure 12. Energy levels (shown as horizontal lines in ascending order)

The term used for effect on biological tissue that any form of electromagnetic radiation induces is called 'relative biological effectiveness' (rbe). The higher up the electromagnetic spectrum in terms of frequency, the greater the rbe and potential for damage. This is not to say that all is dangerous but over exposure can be at frequencies around the high end of the ultraviolet range and beyond, but long exposure at the lower visible light frequencies may also cause damage. Phototherapy uses frequencies from the blue end of the visible spectrum down to the invisible infrared range. Damage to tissue at this lower range can still occur but now depends on the volume of photons being absorbed and this depends on the source generating the photons.

All photons of whatever frequency originate from electron movements within atoms where electrons, as discussed above, are excited by several artificial methods or natural occurrences. This means everything from fires to fire flies, infrared heat from humans, animals etc. The sun and stars all give out their radiation from within the excited atoms. In terms of phototherapy, there are several methods of producing light artificially for therapeutic applications, covering gas discharge tubes, incandescent lamps, LASERs, gas or solid state and Light Emitting Diodes. These will be covered in the next chapter but understanding methods used to excite electrons within atoms helps to appreciate a common theme.

Light from a flame is the most common and natural example from chemical oxidative processes causing thermal luminescence. Heat causes thermal agitation and is a form of thermally induced vibrational energy. If sufficient heat is present in a combustible material, then atoms will be highly agitated, causing their outer shell electrons to break away, ionising the atom. Other similarly liberated electrons will collide with normal atoms and the energy of the collision will displace electrons in lower energy levels to be further displaced to higher energy ones. In doing so, when returning to their original level, this will release the energy from the collision as photons. These photons will be at frequencies both within and outside of the visible light spectrum. Within the visible part of the spectrum blue flames indicate high energy exchanges whilst red flames are lower. Lower in frequency still, far infrared is also emitted and is sensed as radiant heat. So, from combustion we have photons at different wavelengths being emitted dependent upon the level of excitation. These photons will be widely dispersed in all directions and travel at light speed.

In therapy, our main concern is with electro-thermo-luminescence or electro-luminescence. Both are transductions from an electrical source. Thermo-luminescence is light due to heat, as with the flame example above, and can also be caused by electron collisions being forced along a conductor. Collisions with atoms making up the conductor agitates them causing the release of photons both in the visible wavelength and the deep infrared wave-length as heat. Heat lamps and electric radiators are typical examples of these and heat lamps can be used in therapy, usually in both visible and far infrared ranges. Pure electro-luminescence is caused by several methods. Gas discharge lamps, LASERs, Light emitting diodes are examples of these sources of light and therapeutic phototherapy is largely derived from such sources. Very little heat is involved in the production of photons by these methods, so any effects on tissue are down purely to the absorption of photons within the visible wavelength and perhaps at the fringes of it.

Generically 'Laser' is used as a common term for many light therapies, due to the association with some devices that may contain a pure laser. This term originates from the early design of lasers, referring to the method of stimulation. Modern therapeutic ones are generally solid state and work by generating light from specially treated materials. Older lasers, and to some extent modern ones, especially those requiring very high intensity outputs, still tend to utilise the ionisation of gases as their medium for generating and processing light.

The term laser is also incorrect for many devices used in phototherapy as they do not contain a true laser, and there is much misinformation about them that will be discussed in a later chapter. The next chapter highlights LASER processes and characteristics and investigates the common method of basic light generation, whether a therapy applicator contains a true laser or LED non-laser cluster. Laser is a term that conjures up to some a 'ray gun' type of technology, such that there is an oft-stated belief in some that such technological devices must be superior to lesser powered therapy systems. In chapter six we will investigate such claims. The same sort of logic also applies to the costs. 'The higher the cost the more effective the equipment' does not necessarily ring true, and having some understanding of the technical jargon helps in the selection of devices based on function rather that cost.

Chapter Five

LASERS AND LEDS (IT'S ALL DONE BY MIRRORS!)

Light Amplification by Stimulated Emission of Radiation applies purely to lasers, and light generated by such devices effectively started modern approaches to phototherapy and continues to do so. However, the development of the light emitting diodes in themselves has led to sufficiently bright emitters that can have a therapeutic effect without the inherent dangers of LASERs. Both lasers and LED emitters have their usefulness in therapy, sometimes individually, whilst others within combination applicators. In this chapter, we will look at both types in their construction and application.

Unravelling the mysteries of lasers should lead to the understanding of terminology such as 'temporal cohesion', 'spot density' and 'coherency'. The term 'laser' is often used as a generic term for applying phototherapy. Though technically incorrect for many applicators, it has evolved much like the brand name 'Hoover' to indicate vacuuming regardless of the make of the machine being used. If a manufacturer suggests that an LED device is a laser, then this would be in breach of advertising standards law unless a true laser is embedded in the applicator. The same would be true if a therapist misrepresents treatment specifically as such even though the effectiveness of a non- 'true laser' device is well established.

In the early days of the laser development, various mediums were used to cause ionisation within them. The earliest used a ruby crystal. This ionisation caused the production of photons in a ruby crystal to give out light as they fluoresced. The frequencies given out were in the upper visible red region of the electromagnetic spectrum (about 693nm). Various methods were used to initiate the process and one such method used a shaped ruby crystal. The ruby was very pure and formed into a tube cut specially so that each end was perfectly parallel to the other and highly polished. These flat ends were then silvered such that one was totally reflective and the other semi-reflective. The ruby was placed inside a flash discharge spiral, see Fig. 13 below.

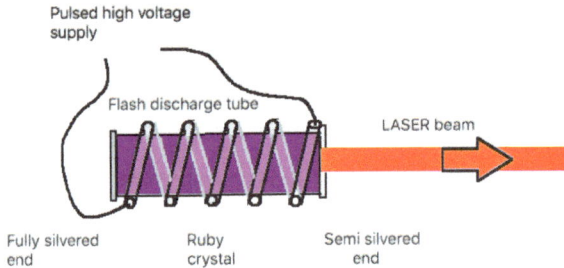

Figure 13. Simplified illustration of a ruby laser assembly

Although shown as being quite large in the diagram, light is emitted from a very much smaller aperture. All true laser devices have the elements as shown above. With the ruby crystal, the very bright flash from the photo discharge tube contained sufficient ultra violet radiation that caused the crystal to fluoresce. The term fluoresce is effectively a transduction of light energy caused by high energy photons emitted from the gas discharge tube. These photons collide with the molecular structure of the ruby crystal, causing electrons to jump from the lower energy states of atoms within that structure to higher ones. As these exited electrons return to their lower energy level a photon of light is generated.

In the short time of the discharge tube flash the process, as described, will have been repeated many trillions of times producing the ruby light that then forms the beam. The light generated from within this is very pure and clear. Some of the photons generated from within the ruby will travel in all directions but some of the photons will be parallel along the tube, being reflected back and forth between the two mirrors and building up until they become so intense that the semi-silvered mirror cannot contain and reflect the volume of photons. These will then pass through. The ruby laser requires the discharge tube to keep flashing for the effect to occur, thus creating a pulsed laser.

The ability of a ruby to fluoresce can be demonstrated with a readily available UV torch emitting at around 395nm. Pointing the torch at a ruby ring, or through the window of a watch that has ruby bearings and a visible mechanism, will cause the jewels to fluoresce and give off red light at around 693nm in the same way as the original laser device but without the 'lasing' effect. Modern lasers are stimulated by 'pumping'. The stimulation method is constantly applied and the photons constantly generated. Generally, the power of the laser output is far less than the pumping supply, due to photons being emitted in all directions. Only the parallel ones form the laser beam.

Solid state lasers usually consist of a specially constructed light emitting diode. This is a specialised form of diode consisting of a bilayer of doped but optically clear silicon.

The silicon starts off as a pure crystal, but has special impurities introduced during the growth phase and therefore are usually termed penta-valent (N type) or tri-valent types (P type). When the two types of silicon are bonded together and an electric charge applied across them, a current will only flow in one direction from the N type into the P type. The lack of electrons in the trivalent doped silicon allows electrons from the pentavalent to combine with these structures in the junction known as the depletion layer. Electrons passing through this depletion layer cause a recombination into the 'holes' of 'P' type impurities, and in doing so release photons at frequencies dependent upon impurities used.

Making these diodes into functioning lasers is achieved in much the same way as with the ruby crystal. The PN junction is enclosed within a structure that has the two sufficiently reflective ends to allow a build-up of photons and then for them to coherently pass through the two ends and in opposite directions. If only one direction of the beam is required at the output end, then a fully silvered coating is applied at the opposite end. Important to the design is the distance between the two mirrors.

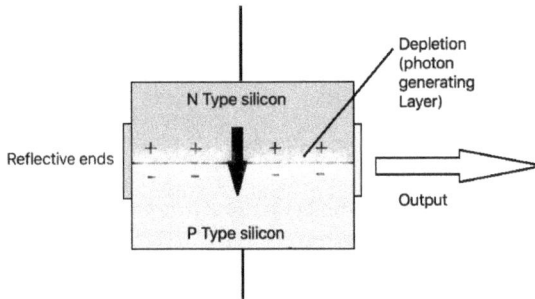

Figure 14. P-N junction LASER diode

For optimum output the distance should be exactly equal to many wavelengths, such that a condition called 'photon resonance' occurs. Figure 15 illustrates this principle. This is sometimes called the 'Fabry-Perot Resonant Cavity'. Photon resonance may have biological equivalence in cellular structures where the dimensions match the photon frequencies being absorbed. This will be discussed in chapter eight.

Of course, many more wavelengths would be between the two reflective opposite faces or mirrors than illustrated, but if properly cut and tuned then a high intensity standing wave would form at the output end.

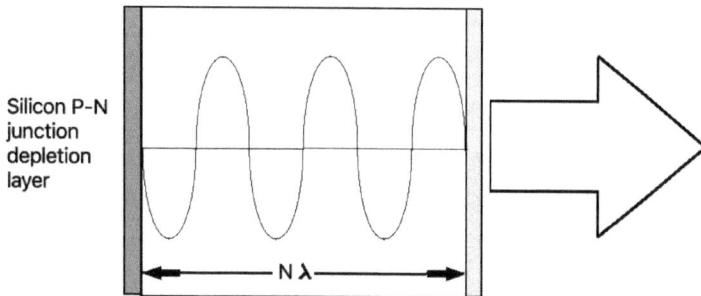

Figure 15. Photon resonance between two mirrors or polished ends forming the Fabry-Perot resonant cavity.

The light emitted has several characteristics. It is collimated and has temporal cohesion losing very little dispersion over great distances. It is also of very pure frequency. The dot formed from a laser when applied to tissue is very small and the next chapter will look at how it disperses in tissue. The temporal cohesion can be visualised as photons in full synchronous with each other, as shown in Figure 16 below. For illustration purpose, the photons are viewed as individual strings of oscillations but may, as previously discussed, be in the form of damped oscillations but still containing the frequency and also still remaining in synchronous.

Photons shown as waves 'instep'

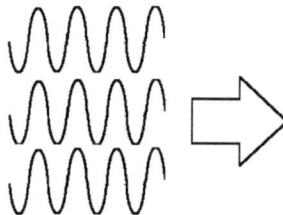

Figure 16. Photons as waves 'in step'.

Because of the inherent dangers that can occur with true laser devices an international standard of classification is used. These currently have classifications in Roman numerals from I to IV:

Class I. This can be applied to all bright light sources including low powered lasers. It does negligible damage to tissue nor causes permanent damage to the eyes if exposed momentarily. However, care should still be taken and safety glasses worn.

Class IIA and IIB These are slightly higher up the energy intensity scale but still will not cause tissue damage. Temporary 'spot' blindness may occur if exposed directly to the eyes. These are used as laser pointers and security devices, when reflected around a protected area. However, blue lasers or light sources can cause retinal damage over a cumulative period of direct exposure. Safety glasses are recommended to be worn if these devices are used in therapy.

Class IIIA and IIIB devices. The intensity of the beam in these classifications is now at levels where short accidental exposure to the eyes may cause permanent damage, so extreme care must be taken with such laser devices. However, short exposure to tissue should not cause permanent damage and can be therapeutic.

Class IV lasers. Until recently, these only had industrial and medical uses as cutting tools and cauterising scalpels and, as such, were not generally considered in therapy.

Recently devices have come on the market claiming to be class IV. The definition of a class IV laser is that it will cause combustion of material such as cloth, damage to tissue and instant blindness if exposed to the eye. These therapeutic ones avoid permanent damage by pulsing a 1 billionth of a second burst into tissue. Even at this short exposure time extreme care must be taken, with all those around wearing appropriate eye protection, including the animal patient. Efficacy of class IV devices is largely anecdotal at the time of writing. They generally operate at around 800 to 990nm. This is well within the infrared range. We will look at some of the claims for all phototherapy devices in the summary at the end of the book.

The heading of this chapter, 'it's all done by mirrors', is certainly true for lasers. However, other sources of light generation utilise parabolic reflectors. Typical of these are the commonly used electric radiators with the heat and light from an electric element focussed forward by the reflector. This is analogous to emitters used in phototherapy that have several common features discussed for true lasers. Modern systems utilise light emitting diodes that generate photons as previously discussed. The difference is that the PN junction generates light when an electric current stimulates the process in the same way as true diode lasers, but it is not focussed and amplified by half-silvered and full-silvered mirrors, and it does not have naturally internally reflective ends as with true lasers. The photons are focussed forward by a small parabolic reflector. This does not produce a collimated beam and its divergence is around 15 to 17 degrees. See photos in figure 17 and figure 17a below.

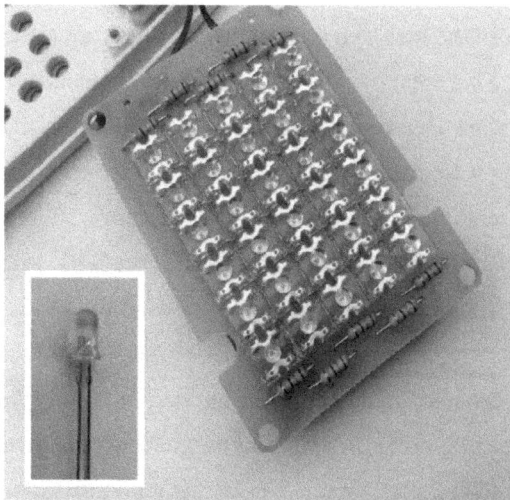

Figure 17. Emitter array used in phototherapy.

When we investigate absorption into tissue in later chapters, a comparison can be made in terms of the distribution of photons from both true laser sources and the non-collimated beams from emitters, but it is important to remember that a photon is a photon, no matter which source it originates from, and the transduction process that takes place in tissue is dependent upon other considerations.

Some LEDs can produce extremely high intensity outputs and the frequency of the photons produced are identical to true lasers, as the same doping techniques are used within the PN junction for all LED sources. Since no temporal cohesion occurs in the light production from an LED source, then a highly concentrated dot is not produced. However, the actual initial light generated at the junction is possibly higher, since the PN junction area of the diode can be made larger and therefore the focussed energy concentrated over a larger area than the spot produced by a true laser. Another consideration is the collective energy of the photons, either at the dot produced by a true laser or the broader dot produced in the immediate vicinity of an emitter.

It is quite often the case that milli-Watt (mW) per square cm rating is given for a true laser. This can be misleading in that the actual spot can be a small fraction of a square cm, therefore to arrive at the actual radiant power this must be divided by 1 cm^2. Take an example of a laser producing a dot of 1mm^2 rated at 50mW/cm^2 then 100mm^2 = 1 cm^2, therefore 50mW/ 100 = the true output power of the laser = 0.5mW. Spot sizes are varied between true laser applicators but when calculating dosage, knowing the Watts per cm^2 value is essential.

The luminescence of LED non-laser emitters is mostly rated in 'candelas' derived from 'candle power'. This is a measure of 1/683watts per steradian referenced at 540THz. A steradian is a mathematical area derived from a spherical object based on the radius, see below:

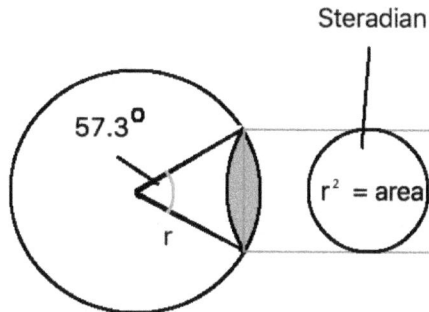

Figure 18. A steradian (radius squared).

If the LED emitter was placed at the centre of the sphere, then the cone of light emitted to cover a circle at the surface of 1 radius^2 would require a conical dispersion angle of 57.3 degrees. 540THz corresponds to the peak colour sensitivity of the eye. An emitter rated at 20000mcd or 20cd would have an emitted luminous intensity of 20 x 1/683 = 0.029 Watts, or 29mW for an output radian angle of 57.3 degrees. Since typical LEDs used in therapy radiate at an angle of 15 to 17 degrees, then their output would be 29 x 15/57.3mW = 7.6mW, or 8.6mW if a 17-degree angle is used. Sometimes LEDs are given an overall power rating, also in mW, typically 15 to 50. This is the total rating of the LED, not just the radiant power, and has several factors to be considered. These factors are:

1. The efficiency, the number of photons projected within the 17-degree cone compared to those generated.

2. The energy dispersed in the direct LED circuit line to reduce the supplied voltage to the operating parameters of the diode.

3. The supportive medium and translucency of the LED mount.

To understand item 2 above, the following diagram illustrates this:

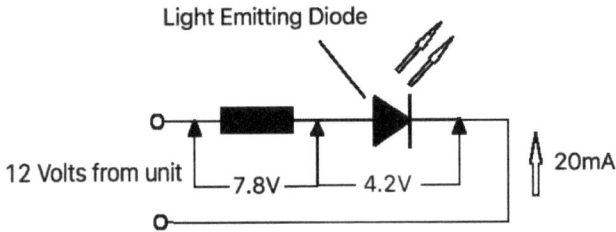

Figure 19. Light emitting diode symbol and circuitry

The forward voltage of a typical blue LED requires 4.2 Volts across it to operate at 20mA. The supply is 12Volts so 7.8 volts has to be dropped across resistor R. The rating as stated is 20mA so R needs to be 7.8/20mA = 390 ohms to limit the current through the LED to stop it burning out. The actual power consumed by the LED is

$P = I \times V = 20mA \times 4.2V = 0.084W$ or 84mW.

The losses in efficiency will come from radiant heat and other losses as mentioned. If the light produced forms a dot immediately at the LED of 0.25 cm^2 (1/4 of cm^2) and if no thermal losses etc. were taken into account, then the rating for that LED would be 84mW/4 = 21mW/cm^2 . In practice about 40% efficiency could be expected, so this then gives about 8.4mW per cm^2 in this example. This is a similar equivalency to that calculated from the candela values. For this emitter resistor combination, there will be heat loss from both the resistor and emitter. 20mA flowing through the resistor will generate 7.8V x 20mA = 156mW + the thermal energy from within the LED itself. If an LED is part of a cluster, then slight warming of the applicator would arise due to this loss.

The above examples are derived from the assumption that the supply is constant. It is more usual to use an electronically generated high frequency pulsed supply with a 50% on-off ratio. This is usually referred to as the 'mark-spaced ratio' (MSR).

Using LEDs in a cluster allows for an overlap between the emitter's outputs when dispersed within tissue, but it should be remembered that the above calculations for both types of phototherapy applicator (pen and cluster) are the theoretical maximums under ideal circumstances.

The additive effect of adjacent LEDs will help provide a higher photon density overlapping within the tissue. See Figure 20.

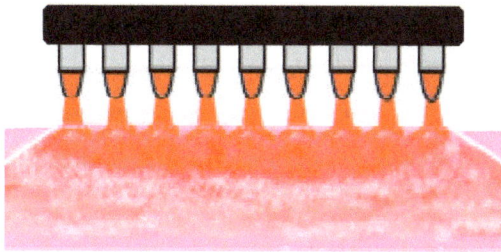

Figure 20. Cluster of SLDs additive effect.

In reality, there are many other factors that can affect the amount of energy transfer to tissue, as well as the depth of penetration at therapeutic levels. The next chapter will investigate absorbance based on frequency within and around the visible spectrum.

Chapter Six.

ABSORPTION CHARACTERISTICS INTO TISSUE

Phototherapy is the transfer of light energy applied to tissue to aid and stimulate the natural repair processes. Understanding the processes involved in relation to how light energy is dispersed in tissue, and the depth that it reaches, is essential for therapists in making informed choices of how to use the modality, and of its limitations. Chapter two discussed the treatment methods and types of injury that may benefit from phototherapy. As stated, no electrotherapy heals. At most, it stimulates natural processes and potentially optimises them. Healing rates are determined by factors within the body and the general health of the patient. Knowledge of depths of absorption and reasoned application of the correct type of applicator is essential for successful outcomes of the wide variety of conditions likely to be encountered. This chapter looks to give an understanding of the basic science involved with tissue interactions and depths of photon penetration.

Any light beams that travel through objects of different densities will undergo refraction. The amount of refraction depends upon the wavelength of the light. This is easily demonstrated by a beam of white light and a prism. White light is effectively light noise, analogous to the hiss heard from an audio noise generator. White noise is, in the audio context, all the frequencies within the audio band that the human ear can perceive and is heard as a loud hiss. With light, light noise is all the frequencies of the visible spectrum from ultraviolet to infrared and beyond. In terms of tissue, the simple experiment of shining a pen torch through fingers, the nose ala or the earlobes shows that the intervening tissue shows as a red glow. If the white light from the torch contains all visible colours, then somehow only the red part of that 'light noise' passes through. In other words, all other coloured components that go to make up white light have been absorbed by the tissue.

Filtering of white light can be seen every day by looking up at the sky. This was alluded to in chapter two in that, providing the sky is clear of clouds, it appears blue due to a phenomenon known as 'Rayleigh Scattering'. Photons of blue light from the sun are easily dispersed when encountering the earth's atmosphere and scattered by diffraction by small particulate matter in the upper atmosphere. At high noon, the sun's white light then gives off a slightly yellowish tinge at ground level through losing a part of its blue component. As the sun begins to set it takes on a red appearance as more of the higher frequency photons emitted from the sun are themselves scattered by passing through more of the atmosphere to the observer. In tissue, visible light is doing the same, filtering out and scattering other colours through denser tissue. Absorption of red photons into tissue is commonly used in therapy. The higher the frequency, the greater the scattering. The efficiency of absorption, in the ideal case, is difficult to measure since much of the light will simply pass through or be reflected. Since red light has been shown to have certain biological effects, then it must be down to only a small proportion of the photons that will be absorbed, the majority being scattered, reflected or simply passing through as discussed above.

In therapy, the three most common phototherapy colours are the blue, visible red and invisible infrared. The most penetrative of the three is the infrared. It stands to reason therefore that blue photons will be quickly scattered at the tissue surface penetrating very superficially, probably within a millimetre beneath the surface. Visible red light will penetrate deeper but undergoes attenuation very quickly down to about 5% within 4 - 5 millimetres. Infrared, the lowest frequency band with the lowest energy per photon, will penetrate deeper but still undergo substantial attenuation within a couple of cm down to about 1% within 8 – 10mm.

Light from LED or LASER beam

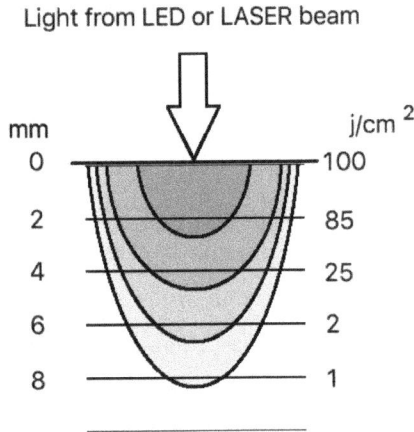

Figure 21. Energy attenuation in tissue (Baxter).

The above diagram assumed an application of 100 Jcm^2 and was measured by Baxter (1993). Other researchers suggest that increasing the power levels does not make a large difference in penetration. Later research by Lars Hode (Tuner and Hode 2002) suggests that substantially increasing the energy levels when measured at a specific distance will only increase the penetration by around 10%. He suggests that the correlation between power levels at the skin surface and depth of penetration is not linear.

If we take the above diagram at the levels specified then doubling the power to 200 J/cm^2 will only increase the depth by between 5% to 10%, Further doubling of power again yields very little extra benefit in terms of depth achieved. Hode states that *"Strong light penetrates deeper than weak. However, twice the power does not mean twice as deep, but maybe 5 - 10% deeper. Let us say that a 100mW laser, at 10 mm depth has certain intensity. If we drive the same laser harder so that it emits*

200mW, the mentioned certain intensity will be found on 10.5 – 11 mm depth and if we increase the power to 400mW, the depth will increase to between 11 and 12 mm." This research suggests that the deeper depths suggested by Hode, compared to Baxter, may be due to more advanced techniques involved than originally available to Baxter. However, other activities within tissue may be at work and these will be discussed in the next chapter.

Pulsing of the beam may increase the number of photons to enter tissue and the depth to which they penetrate. It is further suggested in research by Hode that the wave front of a pulse of light may decrease the surface turbidity and general opacity. This would possibly, in the main, apply to the longer wavelengths.

Looking specifically at blue light phototherapy at wavelengths around 470nm, the depth of penetration of the photons is minimal and can be easily demonstrated by using a single pen style applicator against a finger if it is pressed tightly so that no direct light can escape. Tissue is said to be turbid and of varying density such that dispersion and scattering of photons starts very much at the surface. With this experiment, a ring of blue light will be visible around the tightly pressed applicator forming a circle around the pen extending to around 1mm. If the experiment is repeated with a red pen-applicator, then the area will be illuminated as the tissue allows this frequency of photon to easily penetrate and scatter well beyond the pen's circle.

This simple test illustrates that blue is quickly absorbed and scattered by the underlying tissue, allowing only the very superficially reflected photons more laterally to show very close up and around the applicator. This has significance in how blue light can be used on surface-borne bacteria, especially around open wounds. Photons reflected from a similar sized infrared pen-applicator would penetrate deeper than that from the red applicator but would need a different detection system from the human eye to show this. It could be argued that the ratios of lateral distances absorbed and attenuated to specific energy levels between the blue, red and infrared could be a 'yardstick' indication of the comparative depths of penetration for a tissue type. The parameters would have to be similar and the target tissue identical in each case. However, underlying structures such as tendon and bone and the vascular system may have a significant effect on the reflection and absorption characteristics. In the real-world situation, this would be difficult to measure.

Depth of penetration of the different colours is just one of the factors that should be considered. Photon density is not just directly related to the power of the emitter but the energy per photon as well. If the biological effect on tissue depends upon the energy absorbed by the target tissue, then logically, infrared radiation would need several times more powerful emitters than red, as the photon density would be less due to greater penetration of tissue. Photon for photon, red carries more energy than infrared but is concentrated by being dispersed mainly in the subdermal region where epithelial cell growth takes place. Conversely, infrared may reach beyond the epithelial layers where the energy absorbed would be proportionately less due the energy levels and greater area of absorption and hence lesser photon density. This has implications for timing of application and the biological effectiveness as discussed in chapter two.

Baxter suggests that a therapeutic transfer of between 1 and 3 joules is the ideal amount to be transferred into tissue. This value may be arbitrary but is based on feedback from anecdotal reports and from experiments carried out on various conditions. The main problem with its general use is that no two conditions or depths of injury are the same. Also, the general health of the subject may be a factor in the recovery time. We know that there is an effect beneficial to a range of conditions, and more formal research based upon defined parameters and analysis has been carried out and these will be highlighted in chapter ten.

The time to transfer this amount of energy as suggested by Baxter depends upon many factors, especially with animals. In the ideal situation, application directly on the skin offers the best chance of absorption but even then, transferring specific amounts of energy depends upon other factors, not least of which is the colour of the skin. The skin's albedo may reflect a high percentage of the light, therefore measuring the actual number of photons entering and being absorbed by tissue is difficult to assess. With animals, the problem is further compounded by hair overlying the target area and sometimes a need to shave the area is required. Where open wounds are concerned these do allow absorption directly into the wound and stimulation of directly underlying tissue.

Some manufacturers make claims that their devices may be applied over dressings, suggesting that sufficient photons pass through to be of a therapeutic value. This is a doubtful claim, since all light is blocked by coverings except for the flimsiest types, the exception being sandwich film that can be used to protect the head from contamination. Sunburn on human bodies, leaving light outlines, shows that those areas covered by swimsuits simply block all light including direct ultraviolet rays. Similarly, a parasol will block out all other direct radiation from the sun. To suggest that a somewhat thicker dressing over a wound can still allow photons at the frequencies and energy levels used in therapy could be described as nonsensical. It may be that the covering absorbs the light and slightly heats up. This sort of heat is a transduction into far infrared and is no different from that generated within tissue by normal thermo-biological processes. The dressing itself will block heat loss from tissue, thus raising the temperature anyway by acting as a thermal insulator.

We have already seen that power levels only nominally increase the depth to which the photons reach in tissue and that significantly increasing the power does not proportionately increase the depth. The use of higher power LASERs in the class IV range may increase the depth but again probably significantly less than the power level of the LASER suggests. Add to this the requirement for very short pulses needed to stop tissue burning, then the jury is out at the time of writing as to the efficacy of such devices over more conventional ones.

A good analogy to class IV application, where under normal circumstances tissue damage would occur with prolonged exposure, is a simple candle flame. Placing a hand or finger into or directly above the flame would quickly result in a burn, the severity of which depends upon the length of time exposed. Passing a finger or hand directly through the flame will not result in any injury if moved with sufficient speed. Heat may be felt but no damage to tissue occurs. With phototherapy, burns can occur with over-exposure as with sunburn by prolonged exposure to the sun's ultraviolet radiation. In moderation, sunlight can be beneficial as discussed in chapter one. With phototherapy, the use of very specific wavelengths allows us to concentrate the effectiveness in both energy concentrations and allows also the control of the depth of penetration by selecting the appropriate wavelength.

Different manufacturers argue about the depth to which certain frequencies reach, particularly in the infrared range, and also, whether class IV or Class IIIB are better. In physics, radio frequencies, whether low frequency (LF), high frequency (HF) up to and including ultra-high frequencies (UHF) and above, all have different characteristics of how they can penetrate objects such as buildings or whether they can follow the earth's curvature. The lower the frequency the better the ability to pass through solid objects. The higher the frequency the more quickly is the dispersion and reflections. With sound waves in the human audio range, the same applies. The booming sound from in-car entertainment systems is heard long before the higher frequencies making up the bulk of the music. This is because lower bass frequencies penetrate and pass through the car's structure, whereas the higher ones are largely contained. Both methods of energy transfer have wavelengths inversely proportional to the frequency but related to the medium through which they are transferred. With sound, this depends upon density of the medium, the atmosphere. With radio waves, the speed of transmission is the same as light speed. This is generally constant through all mediums with some minor variations, but referenced to transit through a vacuum. The general rule must be that longer wavelengths penetrate deeper and any suggestion that certain wavelengths, say 808nm, have better penetrating abilities than 908 (both used in therapy) goes against the laws of physics. They may, however, induce greater changes in tissue due to the energy differences, 808nm being higher in effect.

Another aspect is the claims from some manufacturers suggesting that levels of energy transfer into tissue of around 1 to 3 j/cm^2 are 'homeopathic'. This comparison to a largely unproven therapy system is suggesting low levels are totally ineffective with placebo- type results and only high-powered systems should be used. This is misleading as the only difference between higher powered treatments and LILT (low intensity laser or light therapy) is the time taken to deliver therapeutic amounts of energy into tissue, and a fine balance must be struck as to what is of therapeutic value and where the intensity could be considered dangerous. Unfounded claims by manufacturers abound!!

Deep tissue targets may not be reached by the applicator beams directly but there is a possible mechanism that significantly increases the effect down to deeper levels and laterally to the point of application. Higher intensity light radiation can cause electron displacement and thermal agitation in the atoms which make up the molecular structure of cells causing a slight rise in temperature within target tissue. This will then cause lower frequency photons to be generated and allow an onward transmission into deeper and surrounding tissue.

Research reported and attended by the author, at a 2002 conference on phototherapy held at an East London Hospital, presented the effect on shingles sufferers who volunteered for experiments to be carried out on the rashes caused by the condition. Shingles is caused by the Herpes Zoster virus and is related to Chickenpox. The experiment targeted specific areas for treatment focussing on visceral eruptions circled with ink. These patients were examined regularly after treatment with visible red phototherapy using a single LED emitter on the circled areas. The results reported showed a quick clear-up rate for the treated spots and for those near, but untreated, to the targeted ones. The suggestion here is that other factors may be at work that may allow an area far larger that the targeted one to be affected. This has been described as a photo-chemical effect or a 'cascade' effect, and will be discussed later. Other factors may be photon-reflection, causing wide dispersion especially at the red to blue wavelengths. This may suggest that photons are not absorbed by all structures but reflected off cellular structures, perhaps laterally and down to deeper levels.

Another aspect to consider is polarisation of the light from the applicator. The concept of polarised light may, for many, be difficult to perceive but can be compared with radio transmission frequencies and how aerials are oriented for both transmission and reception. A transmitter aerial that is used horizontally, as with many television transmitters, requires that the receiving aerial on houses and buildings should also be horizontal. These transmissions are said to be 'horizontally polarised'. The same applies to vertically aligned transmitter and receiver aerials but termed 'vertical polarity'. The strength of the received signal is optimised, provided that the receiver aerial is oriented the same. Also, the dimension of the aerials must be closely matched to the transmitter aerial dimensions. See Fig. 22.

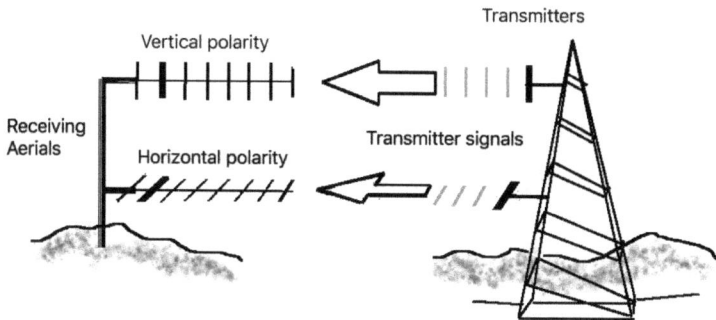

Figure 22. Example of horizontal and vertical polarity in radio transmissions.

With photons, their transmission from within molecules depends upon the orientation of the stimulated atoms. Since crystalline structures used in PN junctions (see chapter 5) are perhaps aligned in one orientation, the light photons emitted from them will be polarised in the same orientation. Hence light emitted from all LED sources, including both true lasers and LED emitters, is polarised. The significance of polarisation in tissue may be that molecular structures absorb photons that are aligned to match the polarity of the photons, whereas other structures will either reflect or allow them to pass through them. The effect of the absorbed photons may also be optimised if the structure absorbing them has similar dimensions to the wavelength. This will be discussed in later chapters, particularly in respect of the influence of specific organelles in both cellular structures and bacterium.

Summarising the factors discussed in application of phototherapy may be listed as follows.

1. Depth of penetration of biological tissue depends upon frequency, the longer the wavelength the greater the depth

2. Type of applicator, single point laser/LED or cluster

3. Direct accessibility and reflectivity of the skin surface
4. Depth of the targeted injury
5. Power of the applicator head, though not proportionally effective
6. Pulsed or steady state beams
7. Length of time of application

A simple experiment using a 1 cm x 5 cm x 6 cm thick piece of white soap was used to demonstrate the scattering of red (650nm) and green (530nm) true lasers pens, both rated at 1mW. These were then compared with red and blue emitter pens (631nm at 7.6mW and 470nm at 4.57mW respectively). The soap could be described as a 'turbid medium', and was used to illustrate similar and even dispersion characteristics for all colours equally. Being white it scatters all frequencies and gives a good comparative measure of beam dispersion. The true laser pen emitters and SLDs were held in close contact at the same point with the medium, to allow a direct comparison between them all. The side of the soap was then viewed for each laser and Super Luminescent Diodes (SLDs) and then photographically recorded. The experiment was then repeated in turn for each pen.

The absorption properties of the soap are probably quite different from the opacity of skin and underlying tissue, although our results suggest that it has a greater translucency than biological tissue. It does, however, have a relatively pure consistency and provides us with a constant medium to compare both the true laser dispersion patterns with that of SLDs and the differing frequencies. The following photographs illustrate absorption into that turbid medium (white soap) from the 4 different sources of light.

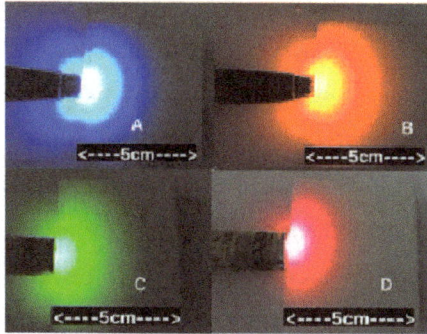

Figure 23. Comparison of laser and LED scatter patterns

A is the blue SLD pen emitting a 470nm beam. There is very dense area of photon distribution at the interface at and just into the surface, extending to around 8mm. The whiteness indicates the high brightness area and the relatively bright light shown at either side of the pen shows a wide dispersion.

B is a 630nm SLD visible red pen. Again, the white and yellow areas just at the interface show where the highest photon density occurs. **C and D** are from a laser pen (capable of delivering either red or green beams) rated at 1mW. If each of these true laser spots are $1mm^2$ then this would equal 100mW cm^2. The highly concentrated dots of both photographs C and D show that the temporal cohesion is almost immediately lost and quickly dispersed. The green (532nm) is more quickly dispersed, as can be seen by the brightness close to the spot source. Comparing this to the red (650nm) is consistent with the wavelength absorption criteria. When comparing the SLDs to the true lasers, frequency can be seen in both cases to confirm absorption and that energy levels play a part in the depth of penetration. However, this experiment cannot be compared as like with like since the SLDs were being pulsed and, over the time of exposure, would show up somewhat less bright than the constantly 'on' true laser pair.

The next series of photographs was taken to compare the penetration of a less turbid medium; clear square amber soap. This was chosen simply to demonstrate beam characteristics over a longer range but in a more visible way. The absorption characteristics of this medium would offer slightly different dispersion rates for the different coloured beams. Yellow is the 'anti colour' of blue and readily absorbs it, yellow glasses are used to protect accidental eye exposure to blue phototherapy. The amber medium being yellowish may disperse the blue more when compared to the other colours but still gives a good comparison.

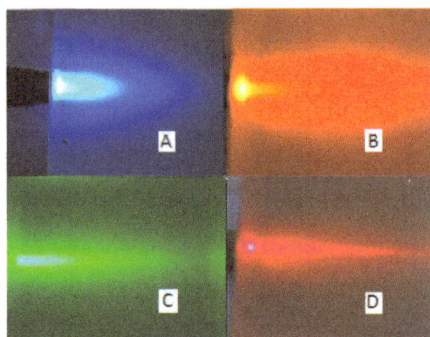

Figure 24. Beam comparisons using a less turbid medium of transparent soap.

In diagram A, the extremely bright area at the interface with the SLD is very small before dispersion significantly attenuates the beam. This may in part be due to the colour of the medium, as discussed, but it also shows a wide dispersion conforming to the theory described earlier. When compared to the visible red SLD (B), where the high photon density extends further into the medium, it can be seen to again widely disperse but less narrowly than the blue.

The comparison with the true laser shows similar characteristics to the SLDs. Unfortunately, a blue true laser was not available at the time of writing but the green laser at 532nm is almost the mid- frequency between the blue and the 650nm red, and should exhibit a greater absorption characteristic than the red. The very bright area at the interface of the green in photograph C quickly disperses into a plume shape. It should be remembered that this light is coming from a very small aperture of approximately 1mm² and is scattered very quickly as it enters the medium. The shape of the scattering is comparable with the shape of the SLD. The visible red true laser beam shown in photograph D has a small area of extreme photon density but extends in a concentrated plume-like form deeper into the medium, as would be expected with the longer wavelength.

This exercise could be greatly improved upon under laboratory conditions where measurements could be taken as the beam is absorbed through biological tissue, but these simple experiments give confirmation of the frequently stated fact that there is little difference in the scattering rates in tissue between true lasers and SLDs. Temporal cohesion from a laser is lost almost instantaneously at the surface. The advantage of true lasers is that they can be held off the skin surface without losing power. The disadvantage is in the inherent danger of eye exposure from reflections and possibly the lack of being able to pulse it. SLDs with their 15 – 17-degree dispersion need to be almost in contact with the skin to gain maximum absorption. If open wounds are to be treated, the possibility of contamination of the pen is a concern. This can be mitigated by using a clear barrier such as cling film (sandwich film) carefully placed over the head and discarded after treatments.

Chapter Seven

THE BASICS OF CELLULAR BIOLOGY

Biology and bacteriology are subjects that require much study. In a book such as this it is only possible to generalise on the commonalities and where possible try to gain an understanding of the potential interactions where phototherapy may play a part in assisting the normal healing mechanisms of the body to function.

To understand how light energy is absorbed and how it affects biological structures, it is important to become familiar with the structure of cells. This is not limited to cells forming normal biological structures but also bacteria, especially surface borne ones that can negatively affect sores and wounds. Eukaryotic cells and prokaryotic cells are different in many ways, with the main difference being that eukaryotic cells are nucleated and reproduce by mitosis, whereas prokaryotic cells mainly reproduce through binary fission. In our first analysis of how phototherapy can affect cells we should look at eukaryotic cells, their typical structure and the organelles contained within them. Later, we will investigate how certain frequencies of light can be beneficial to eukaryotic cells and yet other frequencies detrimental to prokaryotic ones. This chapter will also look at the dimensions of organelles and bacterial structures and speculate about the relationship between size and photon absorption.

In humans and animals, approximately 90% of all cells are made up of prokaryotic bacterial cells (about 100 trillion). These are mainly found within the gut. The remaining, very much larger, eukaryotic 10% make up all other structures or are changed to harder tissue structures such as bone, cartilage and tendons. All soft tissue cells that make up muscle, blood and neural structures are made up of cells bound by a special membrane made up of phospholipid layers in a back-to-back formation. Each phospholipid molecule consists of a hydrophilic phosphor head with fatty acid hydrophobic tails (see Fig. 25 below).

This type of membrane is common to both eukaryotic cells and the inner layer of prokaryotic cells. In eukaryotic cells, it serves to contain the organelles and DNA bearing nucleus allowing easy passage of water whilst keeping out other ionic molecules, with certain exceptions. Special channels allow ionic nutrients into the cell attracted by an electric charge that forms across the membrane. Within the cell cytosol, an in-balance of cationic molecules gives a negative attraction to positively charges molecules in the interstitial fluid exterior to the cell. Not all ionic molecules within the cell are negative, but are sufficient in numbers to allow an overall charge potential difference of around 70 – 140 milli-Volts (mV) across the membrane. The higher membrane potentials are found in the eyes on the rods and cone receptors.

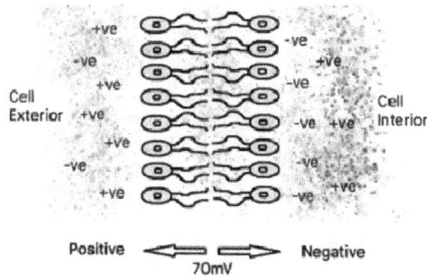

Figure 25. Section of Cell Membrane Phospholipid Bi-Layer Structure

Since the thickness of the membrane is in micro-metres, this small voltage represents a voltage gradient of several million volts per meter. The typical eukaryotic cellular structure has organelles contained by the cell membrane. These organelles are not present in bacterial structures although they do have a similar membrane structure containing their un-nucleated DNA. It is the effect on certain of these organelles and directly on bacterial DNA that phototherapy can either have a possible stimulation or a damaging effect.

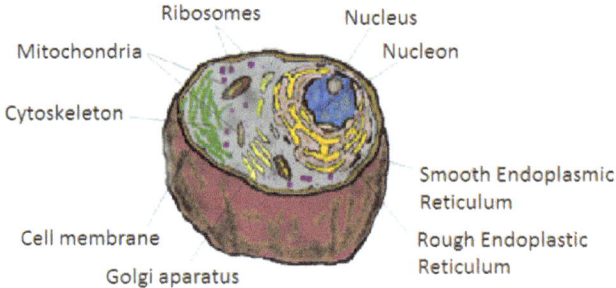

Figure 26. Typical animal prokaryotic cell

Each of the organelles within a eukaryotic cell has a specific function. The following table lists the main functions but is not exhaustive:

Golgi Apparatus	*Assists in the production and modification of proteins. Also produces vesicles containing neural transmitters in neuronal cells.*
Cytoskeleton	*Helps cells keep their shape and support under mechanical stress. Also supports the processes involved in cellular mitosis.*
Mitochondria	*Energy conversion and production. Also involved in the processes involving cell division and death.*
Ribosomes	*Involved in protein production. Links proteins together as instructed by mRNA in the endoplasmic reticulum.*
Nucleon	*Structural membrane containing the nucleus.*
Nucleus	*Largest organelle within a cell and contains cell DNA.*
Smooth Endoplasmic Reticulum	*Production of lipids, detoxification of newly produced proteins.*

Rough Endoplasmic Reticulum	*Rough in appearance due to ribosome attachments. Production of proteins from tRNA at the ribosomes by attaching amino acids with mRNA codon sequences.*

Table 2. Function of organelles within eukaryotic cells.

Organelles containing light-sensitive chloroplasts are only found in plant eukaryotic cells and certain forms of algae. They are 300nm to 600nm in length. Specialised light sensitive organelles do not generally occur in animal eukaryotic cells. However, if we look at specific organelles within a cell and common to all types, then photons affecting cellular processes may be targeted on specific organelles that are dimensionally comparable to the size of specific wavelengths, or multiples of them. This could allow a possible 'photon resonance' cavity effect, like the Fabry-Perot resonant cavity that is essential in laser construction.

In the case of organelles, resonance is from photons originating externally to the structure. Of course, resonant chambers in laser devices allow a rapid build-up of energy to overcome the designed reflectivity of parallel ends. In organelles, the structure is never perfectly aligned so, where some structural alignment randomly occurs, photon reflections and the build-up of standing waves may take longer and be difficult to sustain. However, momentary standing waves may be more prevalent within these structures, sufficient enough to stimulate the organelles' function and provide an increase in energy available. The frequency of the photon may be an important factor in achieving this. Therefore, the dimensions of certain organelles may more efficiently absorb photonic energy with beneficial effects by a build-up of energy leading to becoming resonant as the photons are absorbed. Some molecules such as cyclooxygenase are found within cells and are known as photo receptor molecules, and will be discussed in the next chapter. It has been demonstrated by research that low-level light therapy modulates many biochemical processes, including mitochondrial respiration. Silveira et al (2009) undertook evaluation of this regarding mitochondrial respiratory chain activity in muscle healing in response to LLLT.

Mitochondria are specialised cigar-shaped organelles that are closely and evolutionary related to bacteria They have, like bacteria, their own DNA. Also, like bacteria, they reproduce by binary fission. The main function is that of producing adenosine triphosphate (ATP). ADP gains an extra phosphate ion through a process known as a condensation reaction. This produces a high energy bond effectively storing potential energy. It is then used by the cell, depending on the cell's primary function. By losing this phosphate ion it changes shape to power such things as active cellular transport through specialised cell membrane channels against the voltage gradient. ATP plays a major part in sarcomere contraction in both fast twitch type 1 and slow twitch type 2 muscle cells. Although mitochondria are so small that they can only be viewed by electron microscopes, they number from about twenty to many hundreds, dependant on energy demands of the cell. The physical dimensions of mitochondria fall within bands of equivalent multiple photon wavelengths. Typically, they have a length of around 1 - 2 μm. This translates to 1,000 to 2,000nm.

Visible red phototherapy is known to stimulate epithelial cells just below the dermis. Light frequencies used are around 630 nm. Mitochondria with dimensions of 1.2μm to 1.3μm could form a resonant chamber for 630nm photons. It is quite possible that those cells having organelles that have dimensional lengths directly equivalent to multiples of the wavelength of certain photons will respond more effectively than others. If phototherapy was applied at 630nm, an organelle of length around 1,260nm would resonate as would 1,890nm.

Research suggests that another factor may tie in with the idea of cellular photon resonance, with the concept of a unique mitochondrial oscillator, oscillating at

100Hz, and having the ability to burn fat by way of oxidative phosphorylation. (Alexandratou et al. 2002). This research makes a comparison with a true laser; energy has to build up to a threshold level that allows a beam to pass through its reflective ends. In mitochondria, 'spatiotemporal synchronisation metabolism' depends upon a threshold level of the reactive oxygen species being reached. The rate of build-up and collapse may be a natural process oscillating at a 100Hz cycle. The term oscillator is, in electronics, a specialised circuit that produces a fixed frequency for use further in the circuit. It requires an external source of power to maintain its operation. The theory put forward for photon resonance would indeed build up to a threshold of stimulation, and would take time to become established. The 100Hz may well be the charge and discharge rate of this accumulated energy in the form of physical reverberations that stimulate the burning of fat via oxidative phosphorylation, as described above. It could be postulated that similar effects on other structures of a similar size, such as bacteria, would have the same basis for a range of stimulation processes.

Prokaryotic bacterial cells have similar dimensions to organelles and may similarly respond. Blue light photons used in certain applicators use 470nm and have higher energy than red and infrared. This would possibly resonate, referred to above as spatiotemporal synchronisation within the body of bacteria of dimensions of around 940nm, 1410nm and 1880nm. Since the bacterial cell body contains the DNA throughout its structure, resonance within, causing a rapid build-up of energy, may cause DNA damage and bacterial death.

The effect that photons have on cells has been researched by Moore and Karu (1987), but the mechanism as to why certain frequencies affect cellular structures in different ways has never been fully discussed, only the resulting changes that are largely beneficial.

Chapter Eight

A RESONANCE THEORY OF CELLULAR INTERACTIONS

Before we look at some of the research, I would like to ask the reader to consider the concept that involves the wavelength of the photons impinging on cells and the ability of the cells to discriminate between the different wavelengths and react to specific frequencies. This again could be due to dimensional properties of organelles within the cell and their molecular structures.

The concept of photon resonance discussed above has equivalence, and can be modelled in tuned circuits found in electronic communication devices. In electronic receptor circuits that tune into specific wave lengths of radio transmissions, the circuit should be closely matched to that of the transmitter oscillating circuit producing the transmitted carrier frequency, or it can be a multiple (harmonic) of it. In radio transmissions, picking up of harmonics is termed second channel interference and is undesirable, so measures are taken to filter it out. These types of circuit are found in televisions, radios, radar and any radio frequency detecting circuit.

In physics, the concept of resonant frequencies can be demonstrated by the audio tones from tuning forks, bells, sirens etc. A wine glass can respond to a tone applied close by thus causing it to vibrate as its mechanical resonant frequency is matched. This may result in the glass shattering as the structure becomes violently agitated through absorbing too much energy.

Resonant circuits in electronics can be modelled by an L-C circuit that biologically models the cell's dimensions. This is a coil and capacitor arrangement where the capacitor is charged and discharged through the coil at rates determined by both. The formula: $f_r = 1/2\pi\sqrt{(LC)}$, gives the resonant frequency.

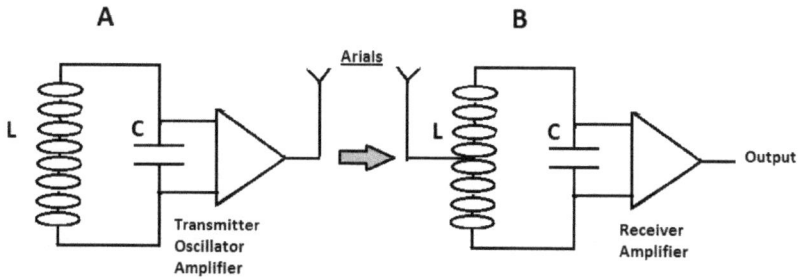

Figure 27. Simplified diagram of a tuned transmitter (A) and receiver (B).

The values of L and C would have to be identical in both transmitter and receiver circuits to fully respond to the transmitted signal's frequency. This also has an equivalency in the mechanical world for pendulum frequencies and can be determined by the formula: $f_r = 1/2\pi\sqrt{(l/g)}$, where l is the length of the pendulum and g the acceleration due to gravity. Both in the tuned circuit example and with the pendulum the frequency is determined by similar formulae: $1/2\pi\sqrt{(y/x)}$. Pendulums physically stimulated by mechanical means will oscillate at only one frequency. A simple analogy is a child's swing. This, being a pendulum of a specific length, will only go back and forth at a set rate when the child is pushed.

Cellular organelle molecular structures may mathematically be described by a similar formula, but the values would be minute and based upon both the mass dimensions and specific alignments of the structure, modelled by certain parameters but only responding to a specific frequency of stimulation. Relating the above to cellular reception of light frequencies requires a little thought about the structure of organelles within cells relating to the frequency of specific photon wavelengths, the effects becoming optimised when certain physical parameters begin to match. This may induce the sort of photon resonance previously discussed within the organelle's structure, induced by the actual frequency of the impinging photons and the harmonic resonant cavity within the physical structure.

To begin to further understand the process we should look at the most selective cells to frequency that are found within the eye. The retina consists of a matrix of rods and cone-shaped photoreceptor cells. The rods, about 120 million per human eye, respond to a wide range of frequencies across the visible spectrum but cannot discriminate any individual colour and in very dark situations provide vision that is generally shades of grey. The cone receptors are less numerous, about 5 to 6 million, and require specific frequencies to stimulate them. They are individually selective to three specific wavelength bandwidths of the red, blue and green colours.

Cones are conical-shaped series of discs like structures that point towards the sclera. These contain long chain molecules of rhodopsin. The neural connections are on the inside of the eye so that coloured photons pass through to be absorbed by the cone. These cause a change in the molecular structure of rhodopsin, termed bleaching, that in turn alters the membrane potential, initiating an action potential that is further processed within the eye. It may be part of the process of generating an action potential that the membrane potential of rods and cones are the highest of any cell in the body and may, by design, require a higher number of photons each to cause changes. Cone membrane potentials may be higher than rods since their sensitivity is lower than the rods, such that at low light levels only the rods function, providing a colourless image.

The above is a simple explanation of what is a complicated process, but is sufficient for this discussion. Cones are said to be pigmented to absorb specific colours and are categorised as S, M and L, these corresponding to short, medium and long wavelength sensitivities.

These three cone types, therefore, absorb blue, green and red wavelengths.

Designations S, M and L that could coincidentally mean small medium and large, therefore the physical dimensions may be effectively 'tuned', being centred on the peak mid-range of the specific photon frequencies (see below). This physical tuning possibly means that the overall dimension of a specific cone has a direct relationship with the wavelength of individual photons. Sizes, in terms of length of cones, are said to range from 0.5µm - 4µm (500nm – 4000nm). Within these dimensions it may be that the actual cones are themselves smaller and more in line with the specific wavelengths such that the photons transduce their energy into altering the rhodopsin molecules far more effectively by this physical tuning and, like all tuned circuits both physical and electronic, will have bandwidth that may overlap an adjacent channel or cone receptor.

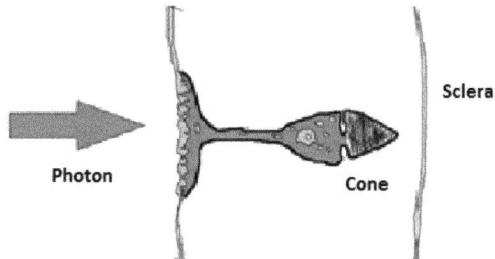

Figure 28. Simplified optical cone cell

The conical shape may well be a focusing mechanism by design, to capture and optimise photon absorption.

Cone	Frequency range	Peak sensitivity
S	400-500nm	420-440nm
M	450-630nm	534-555nm
L	500-700nm	564-580nm

Table 4. Comparative frequency sensitivities for the three types of cone cell.

The above discussion on cells of the eye that are specifically designed to be photo sensitive may have relevance to the dimensional characteristics of other animal soft tissue as discussed earlier. The absorption of higher frequency photons in the blue range may directly impact on much smaller bacterial cells.

In earlier chapters, we have touched on prokaryotic cells and possible negative effects. In the gut, bacteria, also known as flora, can be classified into three types: good bacteria, opportunistic bacteria and bad bacteria. Good bacteria aid digestion by the production of acids, sometimes aided by opportunistic bacteria. Bad bacteria, a cause in many digestive illnesses, again can be assisted by opportunistic ones. Bacteria, whether good or bad, can be problematic if found outside of the gut environment. Bacteria can simply be physically categorised as long, tubular in appearance (bacillus), or rounded and of the coccus grouping, some being almost spherical in appearance. Typical of these is staphylococcus aureus.

Coccus, indicating the rounded shape, can be the cause of many health problems, particularly in humans, MRSA being just one of them. With both humans and animals, gingivalis bacteria are a cause of gum disease. The list is extremely large and the subject of much study, but for our purposes we need to look at material structure and dimensions to begin to understand the processes that are involved in treating bacterial infections with light.

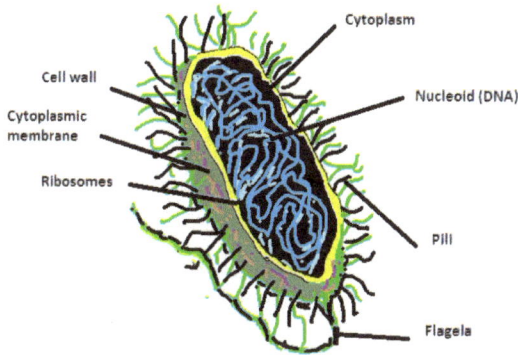

Figure 29. Prokaryotic bacterial cellular structure

The most obvious difference between eukaryotic and prokaryotic cells is that in prokaryotic ones there is a lack of organelles that are contained within the structure. Energy in the form of ATP comes from glycolysis resulting from cyclo c oxidase processes as there are no specific mitochondria to carry out the function in bacteria, and as bacteria and mitochondria have common origins they produce cyclo oxygenase and other processes in the same way. Bacterial DNA, like mitochondrial DNA, is not confined to a specific nucleus either. It is spread through the bacterial body (see Fig. 29).

The effect of light on bacteria has an evolutionary history. In the Pre-Cambrian time of around 560 million years ago the atmosphere was thought to stabilise and remain much as it is today. A light filtering process called Rayleigh Scattering was discussed in a previous chapter. This scattering process filtered out the higher frequencies of visible light, particularly in the blue band. The onset of this filtering coincided with the development of blue-green algae (cyanobacteria) as one of the earliest lifeforms, called stromatolites. These ancient fossils were found in rock formations from that period. It was postulated by the author and others several decades ago that blue light photons inhibited bacterial proliferation levels until the atmosphere became stabilised and filtered them sufficiently down to levels which then allowed bacteria to multiply and evolve.

The common link between blue light wavelength of between 400nm and 500nm and bacteria may once again be a size relationship in that the physical dimensions of some bacteria may match the wavelengths or be a multiple of it, forming a resonant chamber. Skin borne bacteria such as the staphylococcus species have dimensions of between 0.5µm and 1.5µm. This translates to 500 to 1500nm. The frequency of blue light has wavelengths that are similar in length to these dimensions or low multiples of them, being between 400 to 500nm, and would sit closely to this range with internal dimensions laterally well within it.

Bacteria can be found everywhere, both within and outside of the body. Most surface bacteria are harmless and live on skin, for instance the staphylococcus species. Where skin is damaged then some bacteria can invade the wound and cause infections. It could be postulated that natural sunlight has sufficient blue light to have a moderating effect, naturally limiting the spread of bacteria on humans where direct exposure is allowed. However, with very low direct skin exposure on animals, certain other bacterial species will live on the skin and in the hair follicles. It is known that propionibacteria are hair follicle-based and a possible cause of acne in humans, and may be the cause of irritation and similar problems in animals. There are many staphylococcus aureus bacteria that can cause a variety of infections, including furunculosis and abscesses. An animal furunculosis case is listed in the case history appendix, where antibiotics have little effect but the condition was helped to be resolved by phototherapy.

The mechanisms of how blue light may affect bacteria may be analogous to the wine glass example mentioned earlier in the chapter. Stimulated by a sonic tone at the glass's mechanical resonant frequency, the glass would initially begin to vibrate then eventually shatter if the intensity of the tone is sufficiently increased. In a similar way, electromagnetic energy in the form of photons absorbed by bacteria would resonate within the structure containing the DNA strand. Blue light has more energy per photon than visible red or infrared and, along with the ultraviolet that was eventually used in Finsen's anti-bacterial research, base pair damage may be caused in the DNA double helix structure by interfering with the molecular structures and effectively shattering them as standing waves build up.

In magnetism, a magnetic field is caused by the orderly movement of electrons and is formed at right angles to the flow. As a result, only when the flow of electrons is interrupted or quickly reduced is the magnetic field caused to rapidly change in intensity. Only this field dynamism can affect a transfer of energy by inducing a charge at right angles into a secondary medium, i.e. tissue. Electromagnetic energy in a photon is derived from within atoms caused by an almost light speed exchange between energy levels. The effect of this is to cause a release of extremely dynamic electromagnetic energy at very high frequencies, as discussed in chapter four. This highly dynamic energy, released as a photon, has three possible characteristics, two of these being the frequency and amplitude, the other the transit speed, the speed of light. The frequency induction effect would be at right angles to the transit speed. If sufficient exposure arises, displacement of electrons within molecular structures will occur. Photon resonance and the build-up of standing waves within a bacterial structure could be the cause of such damage and hence kill the cell.

The reason why both prokaryotic and eukaryotic cells may be damaged by high energy photons can be related to normal induction processes. With electromagnetic induction, electrons in the secondary medium are caused to react to the dynamic electromagnetic field by repulsion. A simplified explanation of this is that as the field is itself a product of dynamic electrons, it therefore directly affects other electrons, both free and within molecular structures, that the field encounters. If the same principle is applied to photons, then they will naturally affect electrons within structures, because the photon is also a product of energy released from highly dynamic electrons. The energy absorbed from photons will, in effect, also directly energise the electrons they encounter. This could be by causing those electrons that are bonding to vibrate and eventually to damage the bonds. These could occur to both co-valent and ionic bonding of molecules. The effect may result in damage by directly causing the breakdown of bonds, thereby altering the molecular structures.

High energy from both highly dynamic magnetic fields (high frequency, not the low frequency used in pulsed magnetic therapy) and high energy photons can both produce similar tissue radiation damage. Fortunately, with phototherapy, photon frequencies are not instantly damaging to cellular structures under normal circumstances, except for the eyes. This depends upon accidental exposure and the class of phototherapy being used, class II or III. Changes to tissue are additive over the time taken to transfer energy and a gradual effect on targeted structure may be therapeutic before an overload may occur.

Bacteria being directly exposed to a high density, higher energy photon source, as with blue light, may rapidly build up energy due to the resonance previously suggested. Damage may occur throughout the DNA structure as prokaryotic cells spread their DNA throughout the bacterial cell. This build-up of photon energy may be explained using the idea given in an earlier chapter, whereby a comparison of the numbers of grains of sand on beaches was made to the number of photons in just one joule of energy.

This almost inconceivably large number concentrated in a small area would mean that billions of photons are impinging on molecular structures in an almost constant stream. Since the energy in each photon is very low, no damage occurs under moderate exposure and is quickly absorbed and dispersed. The structural resonance concept would provide for each photon to add to the energy of the previous one and quickly establish some affect that, initially, may be therapeutic.

Photon resonance within bacterial or mitochondrial structures would cause a build-up and collapse of standing waves. The rate of the build-up and collapse may be related to the '100 Hz Unique mitochondrial oscillator' previously discussed. When a threshold of energy of the standing waves is reached, damage or molecular transformations would occur, as highlighted in the processes previously referred to earlier. These standing waves would be equivalent to cavitation when using ultrasound, where an additive effect of ultrasound energy being reflected off tissue interfaces causes the formation of large bubbles that then collapse and, in doing so, damage tissue structures. This is termed unstable cavitation. Stable cavitation is the formation of small bubbles almost as soon as the ultrasound enters tissue, and is thought to be therapeutic. This analogy, although totally different in application, is on a similar principle such that lower energy applications of phototherapy are beneficial; it is only when energy levels reach a threshold that standing waves of electromagnetic energy would accumulate to damaging levels.

Chapter Nine

RESEARCH

The British Association of Dermatologists identifies only three types of phototherapy treatments: UVA, UVB and UVC. These are used in therapy for such conditions as eczema, psoriasis and other inflammatory diseases. Qualified nurses and physiotherapists trained as phototherapists, and working under the direction of a consultant dermatologist, are the only ones allowed to apply it. Research has been largely confined to using ultraviolet wavelengths to provide the basis for treatment regimes in hospitals. For the veterinary physiotherapist, training is largely limited to courses provided by manufacturers, slanted very much towards their own equipment, or included as part of the curriculum in accredited university courses. Since the main use by veterinary physiotherapists is likely to be limited to visible light or infrared, finding research within these wavelengths is limited. However, over the last three decades low frequency phototherapy has become more accepted in both the human medical professions and in veterinary professions.

In scientific research, a scientist has necessarily to concentrate on a small area to thoroughly understand part of a process and add to the body of knowledge. In my own research, I looked at one small part of orthopaedic problems and injuries, approaching my own area of study from a different point of view to others that had gone before me. Although I gained a large amount of knowledge from my own studies, I would in no way describe myself as an orthopaedics expert. In looking at the research carried out in the field of phototherapeutics, there are many researchers contributing to the overall subject, although there is no one expert for the whole subject regarding using light in therapy. Disseminating that which is useful to the therapist to the purely academic is a never-ending task. In this chapter, some research findings will be highlighted to give credence to certain aspects of the therapy discussed so far, but it is not exhaustive.

This book has up to this point been based upon much reported use of phototherapy and some of the science and theories underpinning it. Research is somewhat limited, possibly due to the relatively short period of time from the late 60s to the present that it has gained any credibility as a useful treatment modality, based largely on using ultraviolet radiation. With visible light and infrared phototherapy, anecdotal evidence for any device's efficacy is a difficult area in terms of scientific acceptance. Many devices sold as aids to the body's repair do not have any credence as far as empirical research is concerned. Claims based upon pseudoscientific jargon may impress some people looking for answers to sometimes impossible situations of health, both for themselves and their pets. If any natural improvement should occur, it is human nature to look for an explanation and give undeserved credit to some alternatives. However, some research is now being carried out with lower frequency phototherapy that backs up the many anecdotal reports of positive outcomes.

Starting with our own limited research and referenced to myself, a trial was carried out for us by a post-graduate student. She was given the task of comparing the effect of red and blue light on culture plates on which typical skin surface-borne bacteria such as staphylococcus and e-coli were growing. The criteria set was to examine not just different light frequencies but differing rates of pulsing, from constantly on progressing up to 2kHz. The intensity of each light source was constant, but with different photon energies. The wavelengths used were blue 470nm and visible red 650nm.

At this stage, it should be said that the results were not subject to further scrutiny but gave us some credence that backed up the ideas based on prehistoric foundations about the effect of certain frequencies on bacteria. Bacteria (skin surface type) were cultured on agar plates and when the colony was established, mounted red light and blue light pens provided the irradiation sources when placed in close proximity for several minutes using a timed exposure. Control plates provided the comparisons. The results showed that varying the rates of the pulse slowed down growth significantly, arriving with the use of an optimum rate of over 1200Hz. Blue light was more effective than red but both reduced the rate of growth, as did a constantly applied irradiation to some lesser extent. Since this project was part of an investigative report that was not published, then its scientific value is questionable. It did, however, provide a confirmation of many other reports of the more rapid resolution of open wounds and inhibition of infections following application in practice. Intensities of the LED pens used were about 3000mcd for the red and 1500mcd for the blue. The ones currently used in therapy are significantly more powerful as developments in super-luminescence of LEDs have gathered momentum. Repeating this exercise with the modern emitters may show greater improvements.

This piece of research was only aimed at reducing bacterial invasion and subsequent infection of wounds. The conditions would be almost ideal, since no intervening or overlying tissue attenuated the beams and the areas of peak density of the colonies of bacteria were directly targeted.

Research by Karu et al (starting in 1987) has been carried out over many years and her results formally published. In previous chapters it has been stated that the cellular organelles, such as mitochondria, appear to be specifically targeted. The theory of photon resonance within this specific organelle, and also the re-emission of lower frequency photons initiating cascade reactions, seem to be borne out by Karu's work. Mitochondria are responsible for the production of adenosine triphosphate and, when subjected to red light phototherapy, appear to show an increased output of ATP and calcium ions, both of which are required to power the functions of the body. The enzyme cyclooxygenase (COX) is an enzyme found within the cytosol of animal cells. It is responsible for producing neurotransmitters, called prostanoids, including thromboxane that, along with prostaglandins such as prostacyclin, are released when cellular membranes are accidently ruptured. These neurotransmitters stimulate slow transmission type 'C' sensory nerve endings involved in pain responses. The brain perceives these signals as post-injury chronic pain. Prostanoids are also responsible for inflammatory reactions.

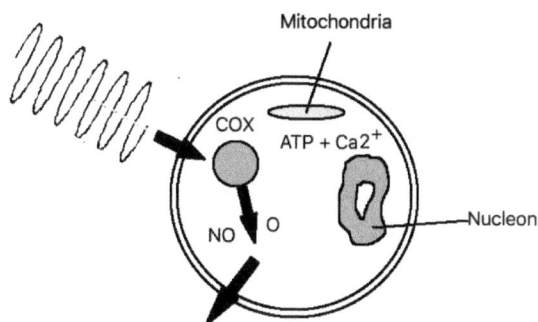

Figure 30. Phototherapy reactions within a cell

Cyclooxygenase (COX) is officially known as prostaglandin-endoperoxide synthase (PTGS). Cyclooxygenase is described by some as the most important molecule responsible for light absorption within a cell, and because of this it is called a photo receptor molecule. The weight of this molecule is 70 to 72 kDa. Da is the symbol for Dalton and is a standard unit of atomic mass equivalent to the mass of one nucleon. So, this size being near or within the wavelengths of photons, is quite large when compared to the mass of a single carbon atom that has a Da of around 12. The complicated structure of the enzyme and structural size may allow photons to directly interact with it, and possibly resonate the structure, causing electron bonds to break. This inhibits the production of prostaglandin, releasing singlet oxygen (O) and nitrous oxide (NO). The release of NO causes localised vaso-dilation increasing blood flow in the area.

There are peaks and troughs if the range of red light is used through its spectrum up to near infrared. A major peak response was found to be 632nm, that is, coincidentally, a common one used in some SLD applicators. The release of NO is due to it being bound by COX. Photons break (disassociate) the bonds releasing NO. Cyclooxygenase (COX) should not be confused with cytochrome c oxidase, the latter being known as a transmembrane protein complex which is found in prokaryotic bacteria and in the mitochondria of animal eukaryotic cells. In bacteria, it is in the membrane and is involved in establishing transmembrane potentials used by ATP synthase to produce ATP.

In evaluating current and recent research there are many references that can be found on the internet. Relevance to veterinary physiotherapy can be confusing and so is better divided into general areas of research likely to be effective when used in therapy. These are:

- Burns
- Bruises
- Fractures
- Open wounds
- Skin conditions
- Sutured wounds
- Tendon Injuries
- Tumours

The above list is not exhaustive but may cover most injuries likely to be presented to the therapist for treatment.

A Guide to Phototherapy

A search through research papers provides very few references to burns other than to those caused by phototherapy, rather than treated by it. Burns are generally classified as: first, second and third degree. First degree is superficial and mainly confined to the skin surface (epidermis). Second degree burns cause damage to tissue through to the dermis. Third degree burns are those that damage through the skin to underlying tissue and are referred to as full thickness burns. There are somewhat sparse references in advertisements for phototherapy suggesting that blue light has a positive effect on burn injuries and to the use of infrared for deeper burns. I have not generally referenced this as there are inconsistencies in the advertisements and the reference unavailable. Logically, the use of blue light on the burn area should help reduce bacterial infection that appears to be a major problem for deeper injuries.

A few references suggest that phototherapy is an aid for a variety of skin conditions including lesions. Narrowband UVB treatment is used for treating those arising out of overactive immune systems manifested at the skin surface. Much of this type of use may have arisen from the research carried out by Finsen in the 19th century where he later focussed on the use of UV light as a therapy. Current formal phototherapy research is lacking and especially so is research on animals. However, the therapist or veterinary surgeon can extrapolate from human treatments where similarities in conditions between animal and human conditions arise.

Bruises are also poorly researched since their occurrences are very common and in normal situations clear up as the healing process continues at a rate determined by the body. Bruising in animal injuries may be difficult to detect due to skin covering. Where detected, phototherapy, causing the localised production of nitric oxide, may disperse the bruise more quickly and may also assist the resolution of the injury causing it.

Research on the use of phototherapy on tendons has been undertaken on animals, notably rats. Casalechi et al (2013) used 830nm low intensity laser therapy on traumatic Achilles tendon injuries. The animals were euthanised at 7 and 14 days and histological analysis showed a marked reduction in inflammatory cells between the phototherapy treated group and the control group. This research was interesting because a comparison was between 3 groups: 1st untreated, 2nd treated with diclofenac and 3rd with a low powered laser. The analysis suggests that within 7 days the phototherapy treated group presented collagen types I and III in the same proportion. The diclofenac group presented more type III fibres. The research suggests that rupture strength tested after 14 days were the same for both diclofenac and phototherapy. This research, reported in Lasers in Medical Science Publication, is difficult to extrapolate to tendon treatments for larger animals. The main aspects are the size of the subjects, in that very small amounts of tissue cover the target tendons and the type of phototherapy device used. In the range of animals presented to the therapist for treatment, access through hair and tissue may be restrictive. However, using a higher frequency phototherapy device as opposed to the infrared one used may allow a cascade effect to affect tendons.

Other tendon research on larger animals (in this case sheep), again using infrared 890nm non-laser LEDs, has been carried out in Brazil (Lima de Mattos et al. 2015), and this was also reported in the publication 'Lasers in Medical Science'. This involved carrying out partial tenotomies of 0.2cm length in the second third of the superficial digital flexor tendon, in 10 healthy subjects. Two groups were used, one treated and one as a control. The abstract summarising the overall results, reported that biopsies were performed after 28 days. The absence of lameness was reported in the treated group along with sensitivity to pain. It is also reported that significant vascularisation occurred in the treated group, as evidenced when assessed using Doppler ultrasonography. The evolution, rate of healing, of the wounds was not affected but a reduction in the inflammatory response was noted in this group. However, surgically produced tendon lesions are different to those caused by accidents including their nature, diagnosis and analysis. However, the results give a positive view on improvements using infrared LEDs.

In this book, critical analysis of research is not a general feature. Formal critical analysis is part of the process of post graduate students in developing and extending their research based on the finding of others.

Research on wound healing (Eissa et al. 2017) was reported in the publication 'Lasers in Medical Science', regarding utilising a low- powered visible red laser at 632nm, 4mW/cm^2 and was based on investigating to see if it could facilitate wound healing processes in rats with induced diabetes. The rats were injected with alloxan to create this condition. A total of 14 rats were used with a small round lesion created on the dorsum. Phototherapy was applied 5 times a week to half of the subjects and the other half untreated as a control group. Summarising the findings: the wounds in the treated group closed significantly faster than the control group, being completely healed around the 21st day. This compared with the control group whose lesions took between 40 to 60 days to completely resolve. Under these conditions phototherapy reduced the healing time by around half.

The main significant factor in the above research is the frequency, 632nm. This coincides with Karu's research showing a peak effect of NO and calcium production at this wavelength. The use of a true laser as opposed to an LED applicator suggests that a constant beam was applied and that the 1mm^2 spot density was at around 0.04mW (see chapter five, discussion of device ratings). Also, as with the previous report, all treatments were under strict clinically controlled conditions. However, it does serve to confirm that visible red light applied from any bright enough source is therapeutic and confirm the theories and discussions in this book of photon interactions with tissue.

A Guide to Phototherapy

Robert J. Spence and Jill Waible, both medical doctors, writing in an article published by The Phoenix Society for Burn Survivors (2014), reported on the use of 'fractional laser ablation therapy' to reduce burn scars. Although this therapy does not come under the general heading of being therapeutic, it may be of psychological use to boost self confidence in human patients and is included as the presence of scarring on show animals is often a concern. The article describes the process, confined to human patients, where scars arising from deep full thickness burns have left a permanent scar. Full thickness burns require that healing is through the dermis and causes a tight but very visible scar. Most burns likely to be encountered for treatment by the therapist or veterinary nurse will probably be superficial. Ablation therapy is essentially using a higher-powered class IV laser to vaporize fractionally an existing deep scar causing new healing. The new scar is reportedly far less visible. There are no reports at the time of writing applying this form of laser therapy to animals. The term 'fractional laser' refers to specialist devices that emit high energy (class IV) in a matrix of multiple laser dots. These are like a very much lower powered cluster device used therapeutically.

Phototherapy can be used to assist the body to heal both after trauma and conditions arising out of infections. By now the reader should understand how it assists natural processes and reduces bacterial proliferation. It could be argued that any electromagnetic process that indirectly aids healing, by observation and in diagnosis, could be considered as part of phototherapy. Therefore, using photons in other ways, particularly in diagnosis, may be a supplement to more conventional applications.

One area of current research is to use light to allow imaging of subdermal structures, such as the superficial vascular system. University College London (UCL) are currently researching using pulsed red laser light to cause physical changes in red blood cells. Red blood cells appear red because of haems embedded within each of the four polypeptide chains that form haemoglobin molecules. They reflect red light and so give blood its characteristically red appearance. This varies slightly when these haems, that are ionic, bind to oxygen or carbon dioxide as part of the normal blood transport function. Oxygen makes the blood a brighter colour and carbon dioxide darker. This would suggest that oxygenated haemoglobin reflects red light photons more than those bound with carbon dioxide.

Professor Mark Lythgoe, who is leading a research team at UCL (2017), used pulses of red light from a scanning laser to heat up haemoglobin molecules in red blood cells. The research found that this slight increase in temperature causes a minute, but rapid, expansion of the volume of these red blood cells, generating an acoustic pulse. This would be due to the fact that the red photons are absorbed into the molecular structure causing thermal agitation, whilst ionic iron (haems) reflect the photons impinging directly on them. More translucent surrounding tissue is less affected by the laser pulses. Using directional transducers, such as those found in ultrasound imaging, to detect these pulses, an image is built up of the underlying blood vessels. The timing system is coupled to the pulsing of the laser and in some research papers referred to as 'laser- induced ultrasound imaging'.

This ongoing research has great potential for the therapist and it seems to confirm some of my theories of photon resonance within structures that have similar dimensions, close to the wavelengths of the photons. Blood cells have diameters of 6 to 8μm. This equates to 6,000 to 8,000nm. Since red light is in the range of 600 to 700nm, then it may be likely that the blood cell forms a resonant chamber and it is a build-up of standing waves that amplifies the expansion, resulting in an acoustic pulse. If this research results in equipment available and affordable to the therapist, then by examining the blood cells in superficially damaged muscle structures, more precisely targeted phototherapy treatments may be applied.

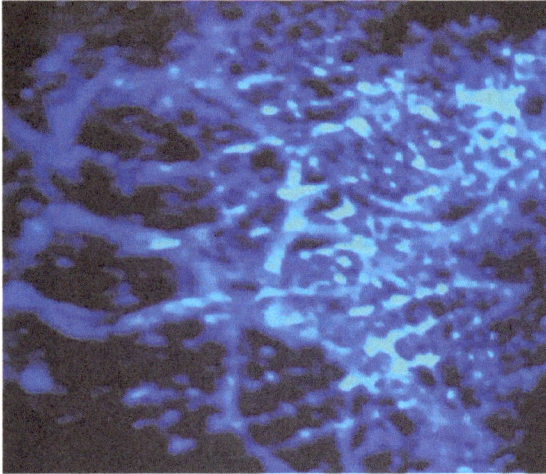

Figure 31. Photoacoustic image showing blood vessels in a human hand. Reproduced by permission of Professor Mark Lythgoe, University College London.

Another form of analysis that may be of use to the therapist is thermal imaging. In early chapters, we highlighted the fact that all bodies, to some extent, both reflect and radiate energy in the form of photons. Some of these radiated photons are in the far infrared wavelengths and can be detected by specialist devices and cameras. Research has been somewhat limited and it finds its use was mainly in industry, by detecting heat losses and overheating elements in both electronics and electrical installations, as well as in physical structures. In recent times, thermal imaging has come into medical analysis in attempting to identify areas of injury not necessarily observable at the skin surface. Since a natural reaction to injury and infections is an increase in blood flow to the area and, with physical trauma, an increase in interstitial fluids, then a localised increase in pressure and temperature ensues. With humans, without a thick covering of hair, it is possible to feel these areas of increased temperature with our own built-in heat detecting sensory nerve endings, but this is limited. With animals, identifying specific areas of deeper injuries is more difficult so a more sensitive method may be useful to therapists. Figure 32 is a thermal image of my dog, Ben, taken in my garden at night.

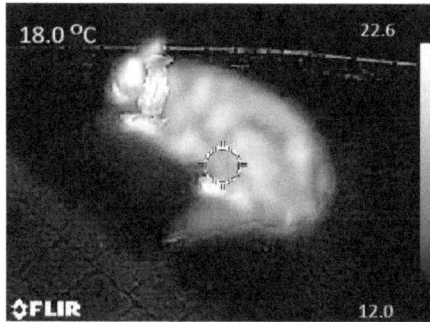

Figure 32. Thermal image of Ben

It is interesting to note that this image highlights several hotspots, and the two visible on his side correspond to the areas of non-malignant fatty lymphomas. The usefulness of this technology may find a place with therapists as an aid to monitoring progress of a subdermal injury or condition. Its use as a diagnostic tool is being developed.

Chapter Ten

CASE HISTORIES

In practical terms, much of reported success in assisting healing may have to take into consideration several factors. These are:

> *a) the natural healing processes and rate of healing expected,*
>
> *b) the condition of the patient and investigating any underlying condition that may affect the rate of healing,*
>
> *c) the nature of the injury or condition being treated.*

Taking these in turn, it is often stated that 70% of all injuries will eventually resolve themselves. The rest are split between those requiring surgical intervention and those that are infected or diseased. However, since no two injuries or conditions are ever identical, a yardstick reference is difficult to achieve and allow an accurate prediction of outcome. Under these conditions, therapists report resolution of injuries that are, in the main, anecdotal. In animal research, where such injuries arise, these must be treated and it is not ethically acceptable to withhold treatment. Well documented case history reports form a volume of knowledge in which similar outcomes for similar injuries and conditions can be compared using the same modality. Also, with the knowledge of interactions of phototherapy taken from established research, assessing the positive likely effects can be postulated.

From reports of success in resolving injuries with phototherapy, I have limited the case histories to those with photographic records of before, in between and, if possible, fully resolved. The latter must be assuming the underlying tissue has healed.

Of the three animal case histories that are included here, two are representative of many similar cases, all following much the same pattern and over similar time frames. The two human ones included are those I have been personally involved with.

The most common injuries to horses occur as tears or rips to skin, both on the legs and body. The healing process usually involves a veterinary surgeon cleaning and stitching up the wound. In most cases nature will take its course; the wound will heal and a scar will be left that will eventually be covered by hair. Cases likely to be referred to the veterinary physiotherapist are those that have not followed the standard pattern due to various causes. These could be categorised as direct infections caused by bacterial invasion into the suture, ripped stitches once again opening the wound, age of the patient and their general health. The first two of these can lead to some necrosis around the wound requiring debridement, removal of the dead tissue, by a veterinary surgeon. Many illustrations of these sort of injuries can be found on the internet. They are the ideal ones for phototherapy treatments.

<u>Case history one:</u> Anal Furunculosis treated with a mixture of blue and red-light phototherapy.

The background to this condition lies with underlying causes and, in the case of animals, certain breeds may be more likely to be affected. In humans, furunculosis is another name for boils and carbuncles, also known as folliculitis arising in hair follicles that become infected. They can also be caused by splinters allowing staphylococcus bacteria to invade, causing a septic mass. This, in turn, causes hard and painful lumps that eventually erupt through the skin. Anal furunculosis, also known as perianal fistulas, has some similarities to human boils but are fundamentally different in that these are localised to the anal area and appear to be largely breed- specific.

German Shepherd dogs are the most common sufferers and the condition is thought to be coupled with an auto immune system deficit. It exhibits as an inflamed chronic condition. This forms fistulas around, but external to, the anal sphincter, resulting in irritation and painful reactions during defaecation, along with other unpleasant side effects. It is a very difficult condition to cure and is usually an ongoing problem requiring drugs and sometimes surgery.

As with boils (furuncles) the main culprit is the staphylococcus aureus bacteria. The following photographs show the condition on a German Shepherd, where it was well established and had failed to respond to more conventional treatment. The veterinary physiotherapist suggested and, after veterinary approval, used blue light phototherapy applied for a single treatment, followed by red light phototherapy. She reports:

"The case was a six-year-old German Shepherd who had already been treated with a variety of medications and phototherapy was the last option before potential surgery". The area was cleaned prior to application and I used blue light, which was followed by an application of red light on each occasion.

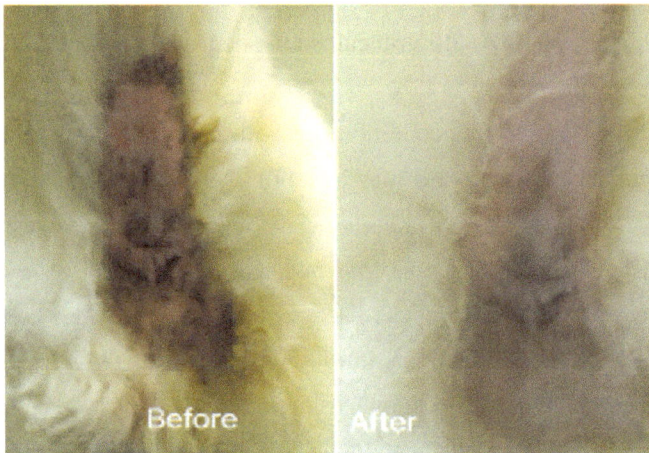

Figure 33. Anal furunculosis before and after treatment

The second of these photographs was taken after the treatment had concluded, in this case one application of blue followed by red, both pulsed at 1400Hz, and shows a complete resolution of the condition. Although this condition is likely to re-occur if it is caused by the dog's immune system malfunctioning, at the time of writing, several months have passed since the photos were presented, no reoccurrence has been reported.

To date, blue light phototherapy has had little reported use for the above condition, but this one is not the first. In 2003 a very experienced veterinary nurse asked my opinion as to whether it would be of any use as a treatment modality for anal furunculosis (AF). I suggested that it might be worth a try. She later reported that she had, with approval, used a blue light pen and had had complete success. Unfortunately, no photographs were taken for comparison of before and after, so I filed it as anecdotal. Perhaps, as more people try it after reading this, then it will become a mainstream treatment modality for AF.

In chapter two of this book, it was suggested that one of the most useful uses of phototherapy is in treating lesions. AF is an unusual, almost breed-specific condition that showed photographic evidence of success. Comparisons with similar injuries untreated may be possible but these reports are few and far between. Reports rely on the experience of the therapist relating back to similar conditions where phototherapy was not an available modality.

Case history two: Equine chest laceration
In writing this book I have been fortunate to have access to the work of a very experienced therapist who ran a charity horse clinic and funded it by producing exquisite porcelain artwork sold in London. Her artistic talents meant that as each horse injury came in she would photograph progress at all stages. Since many of the conditions are similar and the outcome in all cases has been positive, I have included one of the worst cases she had seen and followed

photographically through all stages of healing. over a period of just over two months. This was a case of a horse involved in a car accident that caused a large flap laceration. The sequence of photographs below shows how the wound resolution developed over a period of 12 weeks

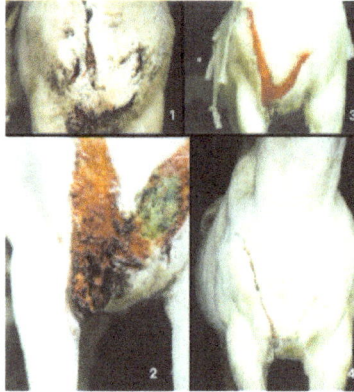

Figure 34. Photographic progress of horse injury after a car accident.

Photo number one was taken after the veterinary surgeon had cleaned up and stitched the wound. Soon afterwards, the stitches did not hold and the wound became open and infected.

At this stage, the horse was sent under veterinary referral to the therapist Mrs Ann Upson who, under veterinary supervision, began treatment of the laceration with red and blue light phototherapy. Photograph number two shows the exposed infected wound early in the treatment process. Photograph number three shows a cleaner, infection-free wound after seven to eight weeks post injury. The final photograph number four was taken 12 weeks post-injury and shows an almost healed condition.

Case history three: Equine leg wound

T G-D, statement:

"The photos should be in date order and you can see that it is still getting worse over a period of a couple of days prior to getting my referral form signed. The horse had received a course of antibiotics that had now been completed and the owner was putting honey on it. Upon the first treatment, I insisted that no more honey was to be put on the cut. - The progress speaks for itself - initially getting worse and then after the application of phototherapy it gets better. Veterinary intervention was a course of antibiotics for the first 4 days and I saw it on day 6 (Jan 10th). The antibiotics were not a tetracycline. The vets were happy with the progress following the start of phototherapy and saw the horse on the 1st of Feb. The cause of the injury was not known for sure but it is believed that the horse caught it on an old tin corrugated roofing sheet that had been blown off a neighbouring property ty bach (outside toilet) or barn roof. The horse made a full recovery and I know he was still being ridden as of a month or so ago".

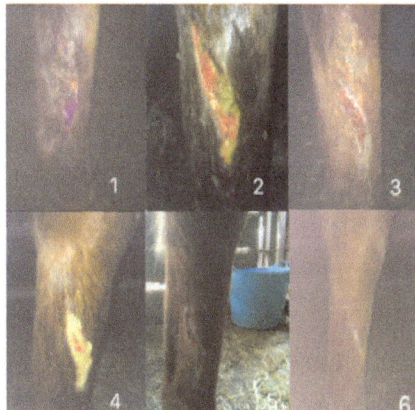

Figure 35. Photographic sequence equine leg wound
copyright to Purple Vet Physio, veterinary physiotherapist Tomas Garbett-Davies
BSc CClinEd(AccMDX) AdvCertVPhys. MIRVAP.

Discussion

Both these and the previous case history number two show a series of photographs taken over similar time intervals. Case number two showed a deterioration of the wound until phototherapy treatment was applied. The rate of healing is set by the animal's own process but may be enhanced by mitigating the possibility of bacterial infection.

A couple of case histories that I have followed through myself are both involving a human patient and one is unique in that a comparison of treatment with and without phototherapy at the same time was possible.

Case history four: Infected surgical sites (human patient)

The patient was diagnosed with oesophageal cancer such that to remove it he would require an operation to remove the cancerous tissue and to lift the stomach to compensate. This required that access be gained both posteriorly, through the lower back as well as the anterior, to gain adequate access. The prognosis given was that without the operation the patient would die within a few months. If the operation was a success, then he could expect another four years. It was successful and seventeen years later at the time of writing he is still alive and in his mid-eighties and leading an active life.

The unusual method of operating left two large sutured sites of roughly equal length. After a short period recovering in hospital he developed an MRSA infection in both healing wounds, more obvious on the rear wound. As this man was a friend and fully aware of my developments with electrotherapies, he asked, on a routine hospital visit, if our phototherapy applicator could be of any help with the developing condition. I recommended both blue and red-light phototherapy. Permission from both the consultant surgeon and medical physics department was granted and application of the therapy started. The rear wound was the most severely infected and the treatment concentrated on that area. Regular treatments were applied by the nursing staff on the back but not on the front. A rapid clear-up rate was noted, to the surprise of all, on the treated wound but not on the front. It was then applied to the front incision and again a rapid recovery was noted. The infection did not return and the patient was soon able to be discharged. The surgeon involved was impressed with the clear-up rate and suggested that it be used in similar cases. This was soon forgotten and no further enquiries were received or treatments given.

Case history five: Surgical sites

I, myself, was the patient and subject of the treatment regime where phototherapy was applied after a triple bypass cardiac operation. As a private pilot, I was diagnosed with blockages of the cardiac artery that required a bypass procedure. This diagnosis came about after a routine aviation medical check-up. The operation went well and recovery was rapid. That was until an incorrect dose of electrolytes was administered that caused the heart to go into fibrillation and spasms. Fortunately, this was quickly sorted but only after greatly concerned staff thought that the cardiac sutures would not hold and if ripped off there would be little or no time to repair. Happily, they didn't and I am still here to write this book.

During a cardiac procedure such as mine, the greater saphenous vein is harvested from the right leg, leaving a long scar from the groin to the ankle. This vein is used for the re-plumbing of the heart along with the mammary artery used as the main one. This scar, being very long, is highly prone to infection and in most of my fellow patients this did occur. In my case my wife brought the phototherapy equipment to the hospital and, with the relevant authorisation, treatment could start on the third day post-operatively. Both red and blue light was used, pulsed at 1400Hz. After several days of treatment, the hospital staff exclaimed that my recovery was many days in advance of that which they had come to expect, no infection occurred and rapid healing soon left a very fine scar. The chest wound above the sternum was similarly treated and quickly recovered. I started exercising my pilots license privileges after 8 weeks post-op. A colleague some time later required similar surgery. He did not use phototherapy treatment to the wounds and ended up back in hospital with a severe infection where the saphenous vein had been removed to the extent that he was unable to walk and his leg was extremely swollen and took longer to recover.

I regarded both human cases as experimental and the outcomes backed up the research findings going as far back as Finsen's initial work. Acceptance within the medical profession seemed slow and with understandable scepticism.

Much of the research into skin conditions suggests that higher frequencies are effective in treating such cases.

General discussion

Phototherapy is one of the choices now available to therapists both in animal treatments and with human patients. Deep injuries are difficult to report on and measuring efficacy also difficult, as no two conditions or patients are alike. Animals present particular problems as the greater majority of them are covered in thick hair. This makes both treatment and analysis of results of treatment difficult. This is not to say that phototherapy has little use over thickly covered areas, but judging the progress of a subdermal condition is very difficult, although there is the option to shave above the affected area. Lesions, however, are where phototherapy comes into its own. It is not necessarily the only electrotherapy available but it is one that can be targeted directly at the problem and the subsequent progress directly observable. The few case histories presented attest to the successful outcomes.

Chapter Eleven

SUMMARY AND CONCLUSIONS

In this book I have theorised about photon absorption into tissue and why certain structures are affected by them more than others. In all my investigations looking at research papers there have been few attempts to explain the processes going on at the molecular level. I have noted that red pigmented cells such as red blood cells do not, in fact, absorb red photons, quite the opposite, but sufficient photons from the incredibly large number directed from the applicator's emitter are absorbed by the polypeptides in haemoglobin to change the size of the structure and result in thermal agitation. Cursory references, by well-known writers on electrotherapies, just make the statements that photons affect the structures of molecules. The theories presented in this book suggest that blood cells, organelles and bacteria have a size commonality and it is the relationship between this size and the wavelength of the photons that focusses and amplifies the absorption of photons within these structures. The rule is 'electrons create photons and as such photons cause reactions in the binding electrons forming molecular structures', often causing displacements in their own parent atoms and releasing yet more photons (cascade effect). Photon resonance theory suggests how this energy build-up occurs in molecular structures. Like all theories at the atomic level, we can only theorise based on cause and effect. Atoms themselves are still a theoretical entity since, up to now, no individual one has ever been directly observed. Scanning electron microscopes have observed molecular crystalline structure in thin film glass. These observations fit in with the theory to the extent that few would ever question the existence of an atom or the structural make-up, including the part played by electrons.

Photon resonance seems to fit in with the theory of selective absorbance allowing beneficial effects to some structures but detrimental to others. Mitochondria in cells largely benefit from photon impingement, since research has shown an increase in the production of ATP. This contrasts with the damage that occurs to bacteria, especially surface-borne types. The experienced therapist knows just how much to apply and on which condition the therapy works. Too little results in no effect, too much is possibly dangerous.

Training in this modality is carried out on some formal courses but mostly in regard to research and the types of injury suitable for it to be applied to. On the course on which I teach, we try to avoid the didactic and involve students in both discussion of theory and demonstrations, delivering training in practical applications for all electrotherapies taught. This enables the student to be not just the therapist when in practice, but also to be sufficiently knowledgeable, to discuss with veterinary surgeons and the more enquiring clients the whys and wherefores of this modality and justify its use.

Most research has been very academic and difficult to relate to in everyday treatment usage, although the more obvious effects of pain reduction and vasodilation have now an explanation from research. It is my hope that those, including non-therapists, who have made it to the end of this book will now look at this therapy in a different light (no pun intended), and hopefully have gained a feel for this modality and understand and be able to discuss interactions with tissue, both research-based and theoretical.

Finally, a word on consideration to selecting equipment. The main constraint may be cost; however, it does not necessarily follow that the higher the cost the better and therefore the more effective the equipment. In my experience, I have been asked to evaluate and repair a device that claimed to be a 'true laser'. It was a battery device that resembled a hairbrush, where the brush head was replaced with four circles of LEDs concentric to the centre of the head.

On opening and examining it, I found that the circuit was a simple flashing one powered by two AA rechargeable batteries. Further examination showed that the LEDs used were in fact standard red ones normally used as panel indicators. Further investigation revealed that the infrared circle of non-visible LEDs had wires to them but were not even connected and the wire endings simply wrapped in clear plastic adhesive tape. This device also had four very dim blue LEDs of little or no value at that intensity. On reading my report, the people marketing this device challenged the maker based on my findings, they then threatened legal action. I offered my support in any court case that may have arisen: nothing ever was heard of either the maker or the threatened court case again. What was even more incredible was the price that this was marketed at £2,000-00. As a qualified electronics engineer, I would have priced the parts making up this device at very much under £10-00 including batteries, LEDs, switching circuit and brush head. Several of these devices had been sold before my involvement.

The above example was not the first encounter with pseudo laser devices. A red pulsing unit was marketed by a well-known company, that again had a cluster of red LEDs in an applicator. The makers recommended that these LEDs were changed annually as they were specialised 'laser diodes'. They were brighter than the true laser device discussed above and may well have had some therapeutic value, but on examination they were not laser diodes but bright indicator types. Again, the emphasis on the term LASER was a misleading marketing ploy and the requirement to change them all annually was totally unnecessary. It must be stated that these devices were marketed in the 90s before veterinary physiotherapy became established as it is today, and the practitioners had little training in both the use and understanding of the devices they purchased, and had to trust the integrity of the device makers.

Advice on selecting equipment is to look at cost, make-up of applicators, energy output as stated, and remember the stated Watts per centimetre^2 is not necessarily the output of a true laser device, but expanded from the small aperture output to a brightness as if the aperture was 1 cm^2. If the device is marketed as a Laser Therapy Unit, ensure that this is correct. Often it is the case that a couple of small true lasers are embedded within a cluster of non-laser LEDs to justify the title 'laser' therapy applicator. This is not to suggest that they do not add to the therapeutic value, but may well add to the cost. Salesmen may well cite research to back up their claims for efficacy of their devices. This is difficult to prove or disprove since research can be only carried out under both clinical and controlled conditions. In this book, I have referred to research carried out by noted scientists; applying their findings into general therapy is difficult since the laboratory is very different to the therapist's application of phototherapy to real life situations and specific injuries.

References and bibliography

I have included many references from various sources, Karu being a major contributor and source. Some of these authors are quoted in this book, others are given here for those who wish to investigate phototherapy as part of deeper study.

....

Alexandratou E., Yova D., Handris P., Kletsas D. and Loukas S. (2002) Human fibroblast alterations induced by low-power laser irradiation at the single cell level using confocal microscopy. Photochem. Photobiol. Sci. 1, 547-552.

Baxter D. (1993) Therapeutic Lasers, Pub: Churchill Livingstone

Baxter D. (2008) Low Intensity Laser Therapy. Chapter 11

Bayer C., Luke G., Emelianov S. (2012) Photoacoustic Imaging for medical diagnostics. NCBI Resources.

Becker R., Selden G. (1985) The Body Electric: Electromagnetism and the Foundations of life. Pub Harper Collins

Bresadola M. (2011) Carlos Matteucci. The legacy of Luigi Galvani. Archives Italiennes de Bologie, 149 (suppli) 3-9

Brunori M. and Chance B., Eds. (1988). Cytochrome Oxidase: Structure, Function and Physiopathology. Ann. N.Y. Acad. Sci., v. 550.

Capaldi R.A. (1990). Structure and function of cytochrome c oxidase: Annu. Rev. Biochem. 59, 569-596.

Eells J., Wong-Riley M.T., VerHoeve, J., Henry M., Buchman E.V., Kane M.P., Gould L.J., Das R., Jett M., Hodgson B.D., Margolis D., and Whelan H.T. (2004). Mitochondrial signal introduction in accelerated wound and retinal healing by near-infrared light therapy: Mitochondrion 4, 559-567.

Eissa M et al: The influence of low-intensity HE-NE laser on the wound healing in diabetic rats: Lasers in Medical Science: August 2017, Vol 32 issue 6, pp1261 -1267. Accessed online May 2017

Finkelstein, Gabriel Ward (2013). *Emil du Bois-Reymond:*

Neuroscience, Self, and Society in Nineteenth-Century Germany. Cambridge, Massachusetts: The MIT Press. p. 272.

Grzybowski, Andrzej; Pietrzak, Krzysztof (2012*)*. "From patient to discoverer-Niels Ryberg Finsen (1860-1904)-the founder of phototherapy in dermatology" (PDF). Clinics in Dermatology. **30** (4): 451–455. PMID 22855977. doi:10.1016/j.clindermatol.2011.11.019

Glennis R. and Ferguson-Miller S. (1995). Structure of cytochrome c oxidase, energy generator of aerobic life: Science 269, 1063-1064.

Hartmann K.M. (1983). Action spectroscopy, in W. Hoppe, W. Lohmann, H. Marke, H. Ziegler (Eds.): The Biophysics, Springer: Heidelberg, Ch. 3.2.7. pp.115-144.

Hug D.N. (1978). The activation of enzymes with light. In: Photochem. Photobiol. Rev. Ed. by K. Smith, New York, London: Plenum Press, vol. 3, pp. 1-33.

Hug D.N. and Hunter Y.K. (1991). Photomodulation of enzymes. J.: Photochem. Photobiol. B: Biol. 10, 3-22.

Hughes M. (1987). Coordination Compounds in Biology. In: Comprehensive Coordination Chemistry. Ed. by G. Wilkinson, R. D. Gilland and J.A. McCleverty, Oxford: Pergamon Press, vol. 6, pp. 541-753.

Jagger J. (2004). Personal reflections on monochromators and action spectra for photoreactivation. J. Photochem. Photobiol. B: Biol. 73, 109-114.

Karu T. (1987) Photobiological fundamentals of low-power laser therapy: IEEE Journal of Quantum Electronics QE23(10);1703-1717

Karu T.I., Pyatibrat L.V., Kolyakov, S.F. and Afanasyeva N.I. (2005). Absorption measurements of a cell monolayer relevant to phototherapy: reduction of cytochrome c oxidase under near IR radiation: Photochem. Photobiol. B: Biol. 81, 98-106.

Karu T.I., Pyatibrat L.V., Kolyakov S.F. and Afanasyeva N.I. (2008). Absorption measurements of cell monolayers relevant to mechanisms of laser phototherapy: reduction or oxidation of cytochrome c oxidase under laser radiation at 632.8 nm: Photomedicine and Laser Surgery, 26 (in the press). 47.

Karu T. (2007). "Ten Lectures on Basic Science of Laser Phototherapy": Prima Books AB, Grangesberg (Sweden).

Karu T.I. and Kolyakov S.F. (2005). Exact action spectra for cellular responses relevant to phototherapy: Photomed. Laser Surg. 23, 355-361.

Karu T.I., Pyatibrat L.V., Kalendo G.S., and Esenaliev R.O. (1996). Effects of monochromatic low-intensity light and laser irradiation on adhesion of HeLa cells in vitro: Lasers Surg. Med., 18, 171-177.

Karu T.I., Kalendo G.S., Letokhov V.S. , Lobko V.V. (1982). Biostimulation of HeLa cells by low intensity visible light. Nuovo Cimento D, 1, 828-840.

Karu T.I., Kalendo G.S., Letokhov V.S., and Lobko V.V. (1984). Biostimulation of HeLa cells by low-intensity visible light. II. Stimulation of DNA and RNA synthesis in a wide spectral range. Nuovo Cimento D, 3, 308-318.

Karu T.I., Kalendo G.S., Letokhov V.S., Lobko V.V. (1984). Biostimulation of HeLa cells by low intensity visible light. III. Stimulation of nucleic acid synthesis in plateau phase cells. Nuovo Cimento D, 3, 319-325.

Karu T.I., Letokhov V.S., Lobko V.V. (1985). Biostimulation of HeLa cells by low-intensity visible light. IV. Dichromatic irradiation. Nuovo Cimento D, 5, 483-496.

Karu T.I. (1987). Photobiological fundamentals of low-power laser therapy: IEEE J. Quantum Electronics, QE-23, 1703-1717.

Karu, T.I. (1988). Molecular mechanism of the therapeutic effect of low-intensity laser radiation: Lasers Life Sci., 2, 53-74.

Karu T., Tiphlova O., Esenaliev R., and Letokhov V. (1994). Two different mechanisms of low-intensity laser photobiological effects on Escherichia coli. J. Photochem. Photobiol. B: Biology, 24, 155-161.

Karu T.I., Afanasyeva N.I. (1995). Cytochrome oxidase as primary photoacceptor for cultured cells in visible and near IR regions.

Karu T.I. (1999). Primary and secondary mechanisms of action of visible-to-near IR radiation on cells. J. Photochem. Photobiol. B: Biology, 49, 1-17.

Karu T., Pyatibrat, L. and Afanasyeva, N. (2004). A novel mitochondrial signaling pathway activated by visible-to-near infrared radiation: Photochem. Photobiol. 80, 366-372.

Karu T.I., Pyatibrat L.V. Kolyakov S.F., and Afanasyeva N.I. (2005). Absorption measurements of a cell monolayer relevant to phototherapy: reduction of cytochrome c oxidase under near IR radiation. Photochem. Photobiol. B: Biol. 81, 98-106.

Karu T. (2008). Mitochondrial signaling in mammalian cells activated by red and near IR radiation: Photochem. Photobiol. 84, 1091-1099.

King P. (1990) Low-level laser therapy: A Review. Physiotherapy Theory & Practice 6 (127-138)

Kitchen S., Partridge C. (1991) A Review of Low-Level Laser Therapy: Physiotherapy 77 (161-168)

Laser Therapy: Clinical Practice & Scientific Background. Grangesberg, Sweden: Prima Books AB

Laser Med Sci. 2014 May;1075-81. 10.1007/s1013-013-1468-1. Epub 2013 Nov 2.

Lewis G. 1926 – Letter published in Nature magazine (Vol. 118, Part 2, December 18, 1926, page 874-875).

Matteucci C., "Sur un phenomene physiologique produit par les muscles en contraction", *Ann. Chim. Phys.* 1842, 6, 339-341

Nam Huynh, Olumide Ogunlade, Edward Zhang, Ben Cox, Paul Beard. (2016) Photoacoustic imaging using an 8-beam Fabry-Perot scanner: Department of Medical Physics and Biomedical Engineering, University College London

Ohshiro T., Calderhead R. (1988) Low-level Laser Therapy: Pub. Wiley & Sons

Pastore D., Greco M., and Passarella S. (2000). Specific helium-neon laser sensitivity of the purified cytochrome c oxidase. Int. J. Rad. Biol. 76, 863-870.

Rich P.R., Moody A.J., and Ingledew W.J. (1992). Detection of near infrared absorption band of ferrohaem a3 in cytochrome c oxidase. FEBS Lett. 305, 171-173.

Schroeder P., Pohl C. Calles C., Marks C., Wild S. and . Krutmann J. (2007). Cellular response to infrared radiation involves retrograde mitochondrial signaling. Free Rad. Biol. Med. 43, 128-135.

Siegel H. Ed. (1971-1981). Metal Ions in Biological Systems: New York, Basel: M. Dekker, v. 1-13.

Silveira et al (2009) Evaluation of mitochondrial respiratory chain activity in muscle healing by low-level laser therapy: Journal of Photobiology B: Biology

Szacilowski K., Macyk W. Drzewiecka-Matuszek A., Brindell M., and Stochel G. (2005) Bioinorganic photochemistry: frontiers and mechanisms: Chem. Rev. 105, 2647-2694.

Spence R, Waible J, (2014) Pub: Phoenix Society for Burn Survivors.

Tiphlova O. and Karu T. (1991). Action of low-intensity laser radiation on *Escherichia coli*: CRC Critical Rev. Biomed. Eng., 18, 387-412.

Tuner J. and Hode L. (2002). Laser Therapy: Clinical Practice & Scientific Background. Grangesberg, Sweden, Prima Books AB.

Tuner J. and Hode L. (2004) The Laser Therapy Handbook: Prima Books AB

Van Breugel H.H.F.I. and Dop Bar P.R. (1992). Power density and exposure time of He-Ne laser irradiation are more important than total energy dose in photo-biomodulation of human fibroblasts in vitro: Laser Surg. Med., 12, 528-537.

Vinck E. et al. (2005). «Evidence of changes in sural nerve conduction mediated by light emitting diode irradiation.": Lasers Med Sci 20(1): 35-40.

Wong-Riley M.T., Bai X., Buchman E. and Whelan H.T. (2001). Light emitting diode treatment reverses the effect of TTX on cytochrome c oxidase in neurons: Neuroreport 12, 3033-3037.

Wilkinson G., Gillard R.D. and McCleverty J.A., Eds. (1987). Comprehensive Coordination Chemistry: Oxford: Pergamon Press, vol. 5

Wong-Riley M.T.T., Liang H.L. Eells J.T., Chance B., Henry M.M., Buchmann E., Kane M., and Whelan H.T (2005)

Photobiomodulation directly benefits primary neurons functionally inactivated by toxins: Role of cytochrome c oxidase: J. Biol. Chem., 280, 4761-4771.